Renal Diet Cool

The Low Sodium, Low Potassium, Low Phosphorus 2021 Cookbook for Beginners. Learn How to Manage your Kidney Disease with the Healthiest and Delicious 250 Recipes

CAMILLE GOODWIN

© Copyright 2021 by CAMILLE GOODWIN- All rights reserved.

This document is geared towards providing exact and reliable information in regards to the topic and issue covered. The publication is sold with the idea that the publisher is not required to render accounting, officially permitted, or otherwise, qualified services. If advice is necessary, legal or professional, a practiced individual in the profession should be ordered.

- From a Declaration of Principles which was accepted and approved equally by a Committee of the American Bar Association and a Committee of Publishers and Associations.

In no way is it legal to reproduce, duplicate, or transmit any part of this document in either electronic means or in printed format. Recording of this publication is strictly prohibited and any storage of this document is not allowed unless with written permission from the publisher. All rights reserved.

The information provided herein is stated to be truthful and consistent, in that any liability, in terms of inattention or otherwise, by any usage or abuse of any policies, processes, or directions contained within is the solitary and utter responsibility of the recipient reader. Under no circumstances will any legal responsibility or blame be held against the publisher for any reparation, damages, or monetary loss due to the information herein, either directly or indirectly.

Respective authors own all copyrights not held by the publisher.

The information herein is offered for informational purposes solely, and is universal as so. The presentation of the information is without contract or any type of guarantee assurance.

The trademarks that are used are without any consent, and the publication of the trademark is without permission or backing by the trademark owner. All trademarks and brands within this book are for clarifying purposes only and are the owned by the owners themselves, not affiliated with this document.

Contents

Introduction 11

Chapter 1: Renal Diet 12

Chapter 2: Delicious Breakfast Recipes for Dialysis Diets 16

    1. Simple Turkey Burritos For Breakfast 16
    2. Blueberry Muffins 17
    3. Stuffed Biscuits 18
    4. Chocolate Pancakes With Moon Pie Filling 19
    5. Homemade Soft Buttermilk Pancakes 20
    6. Cheesesteak Quiche 21
    7. Spicy Tofu Scrambler 22
    8. Southwest Baked Breakfast Egg Cups 23
    9. Mexican Tortilla And Egg Skillet Breakfast 24
    10. Fresh Fruit Compote 24
    11. Burritos with Mexican Sausage and Eggs 25
    12. Orange Flavored Coffee 26
    13. 40-Second Omelet 26
    14. Anytime Energy Bars 27
    15. Apple Bran Muffins 28
    16. Apple Filled Crepes 29
    17. Banana Oat Shake 30
    18. Banana-Apple Smoothie 30
    19. Berrylicious Smoothie 31
    20. Biscuits with Master Mix 31
    21. Bran Breakfast Bars 32
    22. Burritos Rapidos 33
    23. Fresh Fruit Lassi 34
    24. Fruit Bars 34

Chapter 3: Lunch Ideas for Dialysis Diets 36

    1. Lemon Orzo Spring Salad 36
    2. Shrimp Noodle and Chilled Veggie Salad 37

3. Chicken Broccoli Stromboli 38

4. Crispy and Cool Cucumber Salad 39

5. Savory and Smoky Salmon Dip 40

6. Herb-Roasted Chicken Breasts 40

7. Fired-Up Zucchini Burger 41

8. Egg Fried Rice 42

9. Pea Salad and Ginger-Lime Vinaigrette 42

10. Veggie Vindaloo with Naan 43

11. Jalapeño-Lime Burger and Smoked Mozzarella 45

12. Crunchy Quinoa Salad 46

13. Low Salt Macaroni with Cheese 46

14. Chicken Fusilli Salad 47

15. Italian Eggplant Salad 48

16. Chicken Waldorf Salad 49

17. Chicken and Bow-Tie Pasta 50

18. Burritos Rapidos, Fajtas 51

19. Apple Rice Salad 52

20. Beef Barley Soup 52

21. Canned Fish Tacos 53

22. Chicken and Orange Salad Sandwich 54

23. Cowboy Caviar Bean with Rice Salad 54

24. Curry Chicken Salad 55

Chapter 4: Dinner Ideas for Dialysis Diets 57

1. Pesto-Crusted Catfish 57

2. Smokin' Chicken and Mustard Sauce 58

3. Meatloaf 59

4. Grilled Pork Chops and Peach Glaze 60

5. Gnocchi and Chicken Dumplings 61

6. Bourbon Glazed Skirt Steak 62

7. Chicken Pot Pie Stew 63

8. BBQ Baby Back Ribs, Sauce-less 64

9. Roast Pork Loin With Tart and Sweet Apple Stuffing 65

10. Asparagus and Spaghetti Carbonara 66

11. Cabbage, Onion Sweet Pepper Medley 67
12. Adobo Marinated Tilapia Tapas 68
13. Crunchy and Sweet and Coleslaw 69
14. Red Cabbage Casserole 70
15. Mediterranean Green Beans 71
16. Zucchini Saute 72
17. Smothered Pork Chops with Sautéed Greens 72
18. Crunchy Lemon Herbed Chicken 74
19. Orzo Salad 75
20. Chili Cornbread Casserole 76
21. Lemon Chicken, Slow-Cooked 77
22. Green Bean Casserole 78
23. Beef Stroganoff with Egg Noodles 79
24. Slow-Cooked Pulled Pork, Hawaiian-Style 80
25. Herb Crusted Roast Leg of Lamb 81
26. Herb-Crusted Pork Loin 82
27. Black Bean Burger and Cilantro Slaw 83
28. Egg, Bacon, and Shrimp Grit Cakes with Cheese Sauce 84
29. Cranberry Pork Roast 85
30. Bavarian Pot Roast 86
31. Spicy Beef Stir-Fry 87
32. Zesty Orange Tilapia 88
33. Mashed Carrots and Ginger 89
34. Aromatic Herbed Rice 89
35. Sautéed Collard Greens 90
36. Tex Mex Bowl 91
37. Pasta with a Cheesy Meat Sauce 91
38. Rice Pilaf Baked in Pumpkin 92
39. BBQ Ribs with Marinade 94
40. Shrimp and Coconut Curry Noodle Bowl 5 servings 95
41. Curried Turkey with Rice 96
42. Marinated Shrimp 97
43. Honey Garlic Chicken 97
44. Chili Con Carne with Rice 98

45. Honey Mustard Sauce and Chicken Nuggets 99
46. Chicken Enchiladas 99
47. Garlic Shrimp 101
48. Beef Ribs 101
49. Sukiyaki and Rice 102
50. Spicy Pork Chops with Apples 103
51. Shrimp Scampi 104
52. Rosemary Chicken 105
53. Rock Cornish Game Hens and Tarragon 105
54. Red Pepper Roasted Pesto 106
55. Alaska Baked Macaroni with Cheese 107
56. Baked Potato Soup 107
57. Chicken or Beef Enchiladas 108
58. Broccoli Chicken Casserole 109
59. Chicken' N Corn Chowder 109
60. Chicken and Dumplings 110
61. Chicken Seafood Gumbo 111
62. Chicken and Cornbread Stuffing 112
63. Chinese Chicken Salad 114
64. Cider Cream Chicken 114
65. Confetti Chicken and Rice 115
66. Crab Cakes and Lime Ginger Sauce 116
67. Creamy Tuna Twist 117
68. Chili Verde, Crock Pot 117
69. Crock Pot Chicken Chili White 118
70. Dijon Chicken 119
71. Dilled Fish 120
72. Fast Fajitas 120
73. Fast Roast Chicken with Herbs & Lemon 121
74. Fresh Marinara Sauce 122
75. Fruit Vinegar Chicken 123
76. Fruity Chicken Salad 123
77. Grilled Lemon Kebabs (Chicken) 124
78. Honey Herb Glazed Turkey 125

79. Honey Molasses Pork 126

80. Hungarian Goulash 127

81. Potato Soup, Irish Baked 128

82. Italian Meatballs 128

83. Jammin' Jambalaya 129

Chapter 5: Dessert Recipes for Dialysis Diets 131

1. Pumpkin Strudel 131

2. Orange and Cinnamon Biscotti 132

3. Apple Cinnamon Filled Pastries 133

4. Very Berry Bread Pudding 135

5. Sunburst Lemon Bars 136

6. Ginger- Lemon-Coconut Cookies 137

7. Cranberry Fruit Bars, Dried 138

8. Molten Chocolate Mint Brownies 139

9. Cream Cheese Sugar Cookies 139

10. Ice Cream Pumpkin Pie 140

11. Sweet Cherry Cobbler 141

12. Mini pineapple cake 142

13. Dutch Apple Pancake 143

14. Butterscotch Apple Crisp 144

15. Low Sodium Pound Cake 145

16. Apple Cake with Sauce, Cinnamon Yogurt 145

17. Carmel-Filled Butterscotch Cookies 146

18. Spicy Angel Cake 147

19. Easy Fruit Dip 148

20. Crispy Butterscotch Cookies 148

21. Chocolate Covered Strawberries 149

22. Pineapple Cream Cake 150

23. Sugarless Pecan and Raisin Cookies 151

24. Sugar Cookies 151

25. Strawberry Pie 152

26. Spicy Raisin Cookies 153

27. Almond Pecan Caramel Corn 154

28. Apple with Cream Cheese Torte 155
29. Asian Pear Crisp 155
30. Asian Pear Tort 156
31. Blueberry Squares 157
32. Blueberry Whipped Pie 158
33. Caramel Apple Pound Cake 159
34. Caramel Custard 160
35. Carrot Muffins 161
36. Chinese Sponge Cake 162
37. Chocolate Mint Cake 162
38. Chocolate Mocha Cheesecake 163
39. Chocolate Orange Raisin Cookies 164
40. Dessert Pizza 165
41. Pie Crust 166
42. Blueberry-Lemon Parfait 167
43. Fantastic Fudge 167
44. Fried Apples 168

Chapter 6 : Tasty Beverages and Snacks for Dialysis Diets 169

1. Barbecue Turkey Wings 169
2. Chipotle Wings 170
3. Cornbread Muffins and Citrus Honey Butter 171
4. Chocolate Smoothie 171
5. Cucumber Cups with Buffalo Chicken Salad 172
6. Cauliflower Phyllo Cups 173
7. Sweet and Nutty Protein Bars 174
8. Herbed Biscuits 175
9. Heavenly Deviled Eggs 175
10. 60-Sec Salsa 176
11. Alfredo Sauce 177
12. Apple Cup Cider 177
13. Beef Jerky 178
14. Brown Bag Popcorn 179
15. Dilled Cream-Cheese Spread 179

16. Fruit Salsa 180

17. Ginger Cranberry Punch 180

18. Green Tomatillo Salsa... 181

19. Green Tomatoes and Goat Cheese 181

Chapter 7: Sides 183

1. BBQ Asparagus 183

2. BBQ Corn on the Cob 183

3. Low Salt Macaroni and Cheese 184

4. Grilled Vegetables.. 185

5. Cool Coconut Marshmallow Salad 186

6. Cauliflower in Mustard Sauce 186

7. Pineapple Coleslaw 187

8. Acorn Squash Baked with Pineapple... 187

9. Apple & Cherry Chutney 188

10. Asian Pear Salad... 189

11. Basil Oil 190

12. BBQ Rub For Pork or Chicken 190

13. BBQ Winter Squash 191

14. Beet Salad 191

15. Berry Wild Rice Salad... 192

16. Black-Eyed Peas 193

17. Blasted Brussels Sprouts 194

18. Buttermilk Herb Ranch Dressing 195

19. Cajun Seasoning.. 195

20. Chinese Five-Spice Blend 196

21. Citrus Relish.. 196

22. Coleslaw with a Kick 197

23. Collard Greens.. 197

24. Cornbread Muffins... 198

25. Cornichon Pickles, Low Salt 199

26. Creamy Basil Vinaigrette Dressing 200

27. Creamy Pasta Salad 200

28. Creamy Strawberry Snacks 201

29. Curried Kale..201
30. Dilled Carrots...202
31. Easy Chicken Pot Pie...203
32. Easy Deviled Eggs...204
33. Easy Pizza Sauce...204
34. Edamole Spread..205
35. Fajita Flavor Marinade..206
36. Ferocious Barbecue Sauce, Low Sodium..206
37. Fiona's Sauteed Fresh Greens...207
38. Ice and Fire Watermelon Salsa..208
39. Fragrant & Flavorful Basmati Rice..208
40. Fruit & Herb Vinegars...209
41. Fruit Vinegar Salad Dressing...209
42. Garlic-Herb Seasoning...210
43. Gingerbread..211
44. Gobi Curry...211
45. Green Beans with Dried Cranberries and Hazelnuts..212
46. Honey Lemon Dressing..213
47. Hundred Combinations Vinaigrette..213
48. John's BBQ Sauce..214
49. Microwave Lemon Curd...215
50. Oven Blasted Vegetables...215
51. Pancakes with Master Mix...216
52. Pita Wedges..217
53. Quick Dip..217
54. Quick Pesto...218
55. Quick Mushroom Broth..218
56. Healthy Chicken Nuggets..219

Conclusion..220

Introduction

One that is deficient in phosphorous, protein, and sodium is a renal diet. A renal diet often highlights the value of eating high-quality protein and typically limiting liquid.

To decrease the amount of waste in the blood, individuals with impaired kidney function must stick to a kidney or renal diet. Wastes in the blood are produced from liquids and foods that are ingested. As kidney activity is affected, the kidneys do not adequately filter or extract waste. It will adversely influence the electrolyte levels of a patient if excess is left in the blood. By maintaining a kidney diet can help to improve kidney function and delay the progression of kidney failure.

Substances that are essential to screen to support a renal diet are sodium, protein, potassium, and phosphorus. Have a look at our collection of kidney-friendly recipes for a healthy lifestyle.

Chapter 1: Renal Diet

To decrease the amount of waste in the blood, individuals with impaired kidney function must stick to a kidney or renal diet. Wastes in the blood are produced from liquids and foods that are ingested. As kidney activity is affected, the kidneys do not adequately filter or extract waste. It will adversely influence the electrolyte levels of a patient if excess is left in the blood. By maintaining a kidney diet can help to improve kidney function and delay the progression of kidney failure.

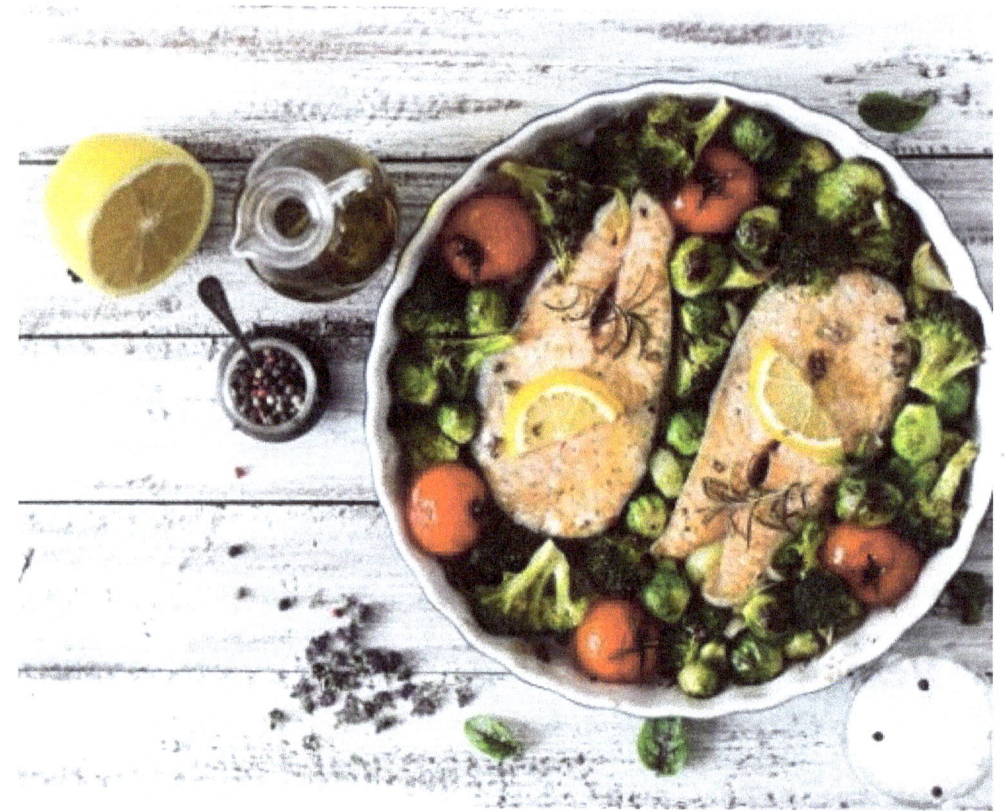

One that is deficient in phosphorous, protein, and sodium is a renal diet. A renal diet often highlights the value of eating high-quality protein and typically limiting liquid. Calcium and potassium will also need to be restricted to specific patients. The body of an individual is different, so each patient needs to collaborate with a renal dietitian to create a diet customized to the patient's needs.

Substances that are essential to screen to support a renal diet are listed below:

Sodium

What is the role of sodium in the body?

In particular natural foods, sodium is a mineral that is present. The majority of individuals think of sodium and salt as synonymous. Salt, though, is, in reality, a sodium and chloride complex. The food we consume may include salt, which
may contain other sources of sodium. Due to added salt, refined foods also produce higher sodium levels.

Sodium is one of the three primary electrolytes of the body (chloride and potassium are the other two). The fluids moving into and out of the tissues and cells of the body are regulated by electrolytes. Sodium contributes to:
- Nerve activity and muscle contraction regulation
- Blood volume and blood pressure control
- Balancing how much fluid is stored or eliminated by the body
- Regulate the acid-base balance of blood

Why should kidney patients control sodium consumption?
For patients with renal failure, too much salt may be dangerous since their kidneys cannot properly remove extra fluid and sodium from the body. As fluid and sodium build up in the bloodstream and tissues, they can cause:
- Edema: swelling in the hands, face, and legs
- Increased thirst
- Shortness of breath: fluid will build up in the lungs, causing it hard to breathe.
- Heart failure: The heart will overwork with extra fluid in the bloodstream, rendering it weak and enlarged.
- High Blood Pressure

How can patients monitor their consumption of sodium?
- To serve sizes, pay careful attention.
- Always read the labeling on food. It always lists the sodium content.
- Choose fresh vegetables and fruits or frozen and canned non-salt-added products.
- Use fresh, as compared to packaged meats.
- Compare brands and those that are lowest in sodium should be used.
- Avoid items that are processed.
- Prepare at home, and do NOT add salt.
- Use spices which do not have "salt" in the title (prefer garlic powder instead of garlic salt
- Restrict the overall sodium level per meal to 400 mg and per snack to 150 mg.

Potassium
What is the role of potassium in the body?
Potassium is a mineral contained in many of the foods that we consume and is naturally found in the body as well. In maintaining the heartbeat regular as well as the muscles functioning properly, potassium plays a major role. For the maintenance of electrolyte and fluid balance in the bloodstream, potassium is also essential. The kidneys help keep one's body's correct amount of potassium and remove excess amounts into the urine.
Why should kidney patients control potassium consumption?

Kidneys can no longer eliminate excess potassium because of kidney failure, so the level of potassium builds up in the body. High blood potassium is known as hyperkalemia, which can trigger:
- An abnormal heart beat
- Weakness in muscles
- Death
- Cardiac attacks
- Slow pulse

How can patients monitor their consumption of potassium?

In certain foods, phosphorus can be identified. Therefore, to better control phosphorus amounts, patients with impaired kidney function may consult with a renal dietician.

Tips for helping to retain phosphorus at healthy levels:
- To serve size, pay close attention
- Know which foods have less phosphorus.
- Eat fresh vegetables and fruits.
- Eat smaller amounts of food that are rich in proteins for snacks and meals.
- Avoid foods that are packaged and contain added phosphorus. On ingredient labels, look for phosphorus, and for words with 'PHOS'.
- Ask the doctor about utilizing phosphate binders at the time of meal.
- Have a food journal

Protein

For healthy kidneys, protein isn't an issue. Protein is usually absorbed and waste products are produced, which are purified by the kidney nephrons. Then, the waste transforms into urine with the aid of additional renal proteins. On the other side, damaged kidneys refuse to eliminate protein waste, and it builds up in the blood.

For Chronic Kidney Disorder patients, adequate protein intake is tricky since the amount varies with each disease level. Protein is necessary for the maintenance of tissues and other bodily roles, but according to the renal dietician or nephrologist, it is essential to consume the prescribed amount for the particular stage of disease.

Fluids

For the patients in the later stages of Kidney Disease, fluid management is essential since regular fluid intake can contribute to fluid build-up in the body that may become harmful. People on dialysis also have reduced flow of urine, so additional fluid in the body will place undue pressure on the lungs and heart of the person.

Based on urinary production and dialysis conditions, the fluid allocation of a patient is measured on an individual basis. Seeking the fluid intake guidelines from your nephrologist/nutritionist is essential.

To monitor the consumption of fluids, patients should:

- Don't drink more than the doctor has prescribed.
- Count all foods melting at room temperature.
- Know the quantity of fluids utilized in cooking.

Chapter 2: Delicious Breakfast Recipes for Dialysis Diets

More than 31 million Americans miss breakfast every day, but you do not need to be one of them. Start your day with a healthy breakfast. It is easy. Eggs are still a perfect choice; they are the safest and most easily accessible protein in existence. Get them to cook, poach, fry, or make an omelet. Put some cheese, tomatoes, spinach, or peppers. Also, make sure to verify the nutritional qualities of the amounts of each ingredient. It is easy and tasty.

Would you need inspiration? If yes, then Check out our other recipes for breakfast below.

1. Simple Turkey Burritos For Breakfast

Want a breakfast that is simple but satisfying? Sauté ground turkey with peppers, spices, and onions; combine with cheese and scrambled eggs. It is simple, quick, and yummy.

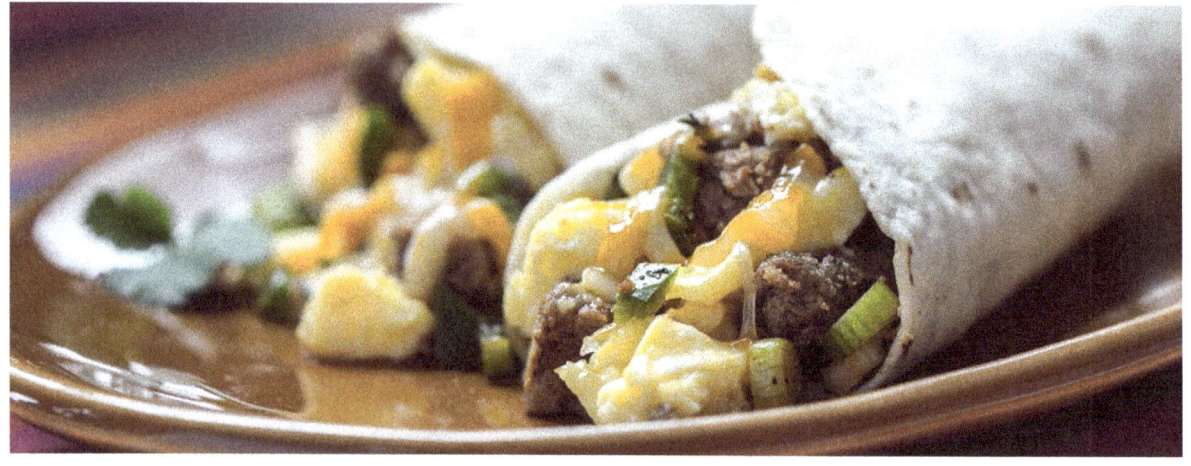

8 servings (1 serving = 1'6-inch burrito)
Ingredients
- 1 lb. of ground turkey or 1 lb. of meatloaf of surplus turkey, diced in small cubes
- 8'6-inch burrito shells of flour
- 8 beaten and scrambled eggs
- ¼ cup canola oil
- ¼ cup diced bell peppers (yellow, green, or red)
- 2 tbsp. jalapeño peppers (seeded)
- ¼ cup diced onions
- 2 tbsp. chopped fresh scallions
- ½ tsp. chili powder
- 2 tbsp. chopped fresh cilantro
- ½ tsp. smoked paprika
- 1 cup shredded Cheddar cheese and Monterey Jack

Nutrition Per Serving

Calories	407 cal
Protein	25 g
Sodium	513 mg
Phosphorus	359 mg
Dietary Fiber	2 g
Potassium	285 mg

Directions
- Sauté the meatloaf, peppers, cilantro, onions, and scallions until translucent in half the liquid. Stir in the spices, then turn the heat off.
- Set the pan over medium-high heat with another broad sauté pan and add the scrambled eggs and remaining oil.
- Place equal quantities of meatloaf mix and vegetables, eggs, and cheese in the burrito shells, then roll and serve.

2. Blueberry Muffins

What would be better than the scent of freshly made blueberry muffins at breakfast fluttering around your house? Enjoying every delightful bite.

12 servings (1 serving = 1 muffin)

Ingredients
- ½ cup butter (unsalted)
- 2 eggs
- 2 cups 1% milk
- 1 ¼ cups sugar
- 2 tsp. baking powder
- 2 cups flour
- ½ tsp. salt
- 2 tsp. sugar (for topping)
- 2 ½ cups blueberries

Nutrition Per Serving

Calories	275 cal
Protein	5 g
Sodium	210 mg
Phosphorus	100 mg
Dietary Fiber	1.3 g
Potassium	121 mg

Directions
- Mix the sugar and margarine until fluffy and creamy, utilizing a mixer at low speed.

- One at a time, add the eggs and stir until mixed.
- Sift the dry ingredients and add milk alternately.
- Mash and stir in 1/2 cup of blueberries by hand. Then add the leftover blueberries and mix them by hand.
- Spray the top of the pan and muffin cups with vegetable oil. Put the muffins cups in a tin.
- In each muffin cup, pile up the muffin mixture. Sprinkle the muffin tops with sugar.
- Bake for 25–30 minutes at 375° F. Before careful removal, cool in the pan for a maximum of 30 minutes.

3. Stuffed Biscuits

Grab a biscuit for breakfast. These delicious biscuits, stuffed with bacon, egg, and cheddar cheese, are great for a Sunday breakfast.

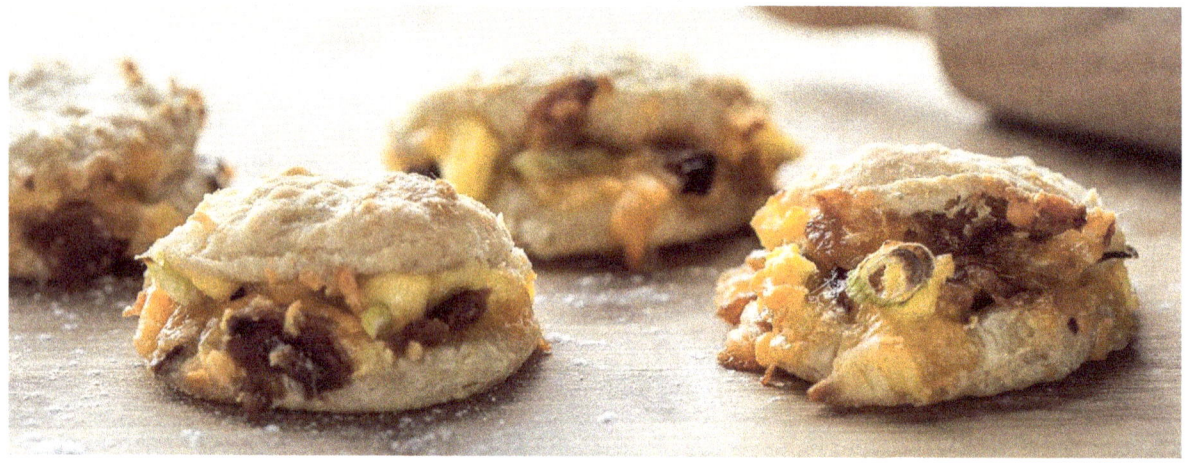

12 Servings (1 serving = 1 biscuit)

Ingredients
- 2 cups flour
- 1/2 tsp. baking soda
- 1 tbsp. sugar or honey
- 1 tbsp. lemon juice
- 3/4 cup milk
- 8 tbsp. unsalted butter

Filling
- 1 cup shredded cheddar cheese
- 8 oz. or 1 1/4 chopped sodium bacon
- 4 eggs
- 1/4 cup scallions (thinly sliced)

Nutrition Per Serving

| Calories | 330 cal |

Protein	11 g
Sodium	329 mg
Phosphorus	170 mg
Dietary Fiber	1 g
Potassium	152 mg

Directions
- Preheat the oven to 425 ° F

Get the filling ready:
- Slightly under-cooked scrambled eggs.
- Get the bacon cooked until crispy.
- Mix and set aside the four ingredients.

Get the dough prepared:
- Combine all of the dried ingredients in a big bowl.
- Slice with a fork or pastry knife the unsalted butter till pea-size or smaller. In the middle of the Mix, make a well and knead in the lemon juice and milk.
- Start preparing muffin tins with a lining or gently grease the bottom and sides with flour.
- Scoop the muffin tins with 1/4 cup of Mix.
- Bake for 10-12 minutes or till golden brown at 425° F.

4. Chocolate Pancakes With Moon Pie Filling

Creamy, rich, and ever so chocolaty packed with 7 grams per serving of protein.
1 dozen chocolate pancakes (4-inch)(1 serving = 1 pancake)

Ingredients
Chocolate Pancakes:
- 3 tbsp. sugar
- 1 cup flour
- ½ tsp. baking soda
- 3 tbsp. cocoa powder (unsweetened)
- 1 egg
- 1 tbsp. lemon juice
- 2 tbsp. canola oil
- 1 cup 2% milk
- 2 tsp. vanilla extract
- 2/3 cup whey protein powder (vanilla) from Body Fortress

Moon Pie Stuffing:
- ¼ cup heavy cream

- 1 tbsp. cocoa powder (unsweetened)
- ½ cup cream of marshmallows
- ½ cup softened cream cheese

Nutrition Per Serving

Calories	194 cal
Protein	7 g
Phosphorus	134 mg
Dietary Fiber	1 g
Potassium	135 mg

Directions
Moon Pie Fillings:
- Beat the heavy cream and cocoa together until they shape stiff peaks.
- Whip for about 1 minute or till well mixed, the marshmallow cream, cream cheese, and whey protein powder, but do not beat it extra. Cover and place it in the refrigerator.

For pancakes:
- In a big bowl, combine all the dry ingredients and set them aside.
- In a medium-size dish, combine all the wet ingredients.
- Slowly fold the dry ingredients into the wet ingredients until they are wet, but do not over-mix.
- Cook the pancakes at medium to 375 ° F on a finely oiled griddle.
- To shape 4-inch pancakes, get about 1/8 batter cup, flipping as they begin to bubble.
- Top the 12 Moon Pie filling pancakes with equal portions; then top those with the remaining 12 pancakes and serve with powdered sugar dusting.

5. Homemade Soft Buttermilk Pancakes

For breakfast, this simple, made from buttermilk pancake recipe will also have you spinning. For a nutritious spin, eat it with fresh berries.

9 servings (1 serving = two 4-inch pancakes)

Ingredients
- 1 tsp. cream of tartar
- 2 cups flour (all-purpose)
- 1½ tsp. baking soda
- 2 cups buttermilk (low-fat)
- 2 tbsp. sugar
- 1 tbsp. canola oil (for cooking) and ¼ cup canola oil

- 2 eggs

Nutrition Per Serving

Calories	217 cal
Protein	6 g
Sodium	330 mg
Phosphorus	100 mg
Dietary Fiber	1 g
Potassium	182 mg

Directions
- Heat a skillet over medium heat.
- In a big bowl, mix the dried ingredients. Add the dry ingredients to the combination of buttermilk, egg, and oil. To mix the dry ingredients till they are thoroughly moist, use a spoon or whisk.
- To grease a pan, use a tbsp. of canola oil. Scrape the pancake mixture into the skillet by using a 1/3-cup measuring cup. Each pancake should be around 4 inches wide to spread. For quick flipping, leave around 2" between the pancakes. Use a spatula to turn pancakes. Do this until any of the bubbles, mostly on the surface of the pancakes, have vanished. Allow its other side to brown, so the middle is no longer wet.
- Turn to the serving dish.
- Think about serving a side of eggs or fresh berries for a healthier twist.

6. Cheesesteak Quiche

6 servings (1 serving = 1/6 cheesesteak quiche)

Ingredients
- 1 cup diced onions
- ½ lb. shaved, coarsely chopped sirloin steak meat
- 2 tbsp. canola oil
- 5 beaten eggs
- ½ cup shredded pepper jack cheese
- 1" x 9" deep prepared piecrust, par-cooked
- ½ tsp. ground black pepper
- 1 cup cream

Nutrition Per Serving

Calories	527 cal
Protein	22 g
Sodium	392 mg

Phosphorus	281 mg
Dietary Fiber	1 g
Potassium	308 mg

Directions
- Cut the shaved sirloin into bits that are coarse.
- In a sauté pan with grease, cook the sliced steak and onions until the steak is browned. Put aside for 10 minutes to cool slightly. Fold the cheese in and let it stay.
- Beat the eggs and cream along with black pepper in a big bowl till thoroughly blended.
- Spread the cheese and steak mixture onto the par-cooked piecrust rim, then spill over the egg mixture on top and bake for at least 30 minutes at 350 ° F.
- Cover the cheesesteak quiche with foil and switch the oven off. Enable the quiche to sit for 10 minutes, then eat.

7. Spicy Tofu Scrambler

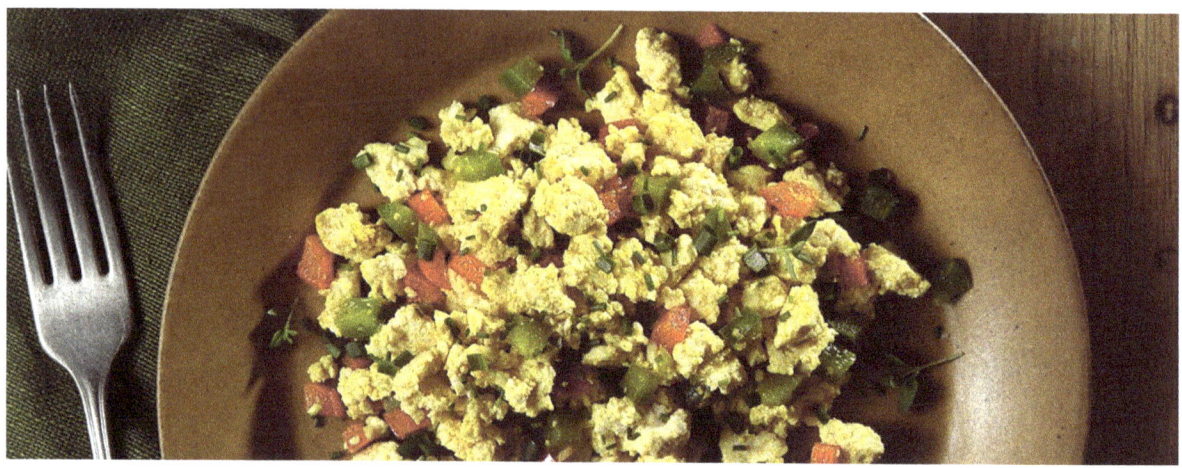

2 servings (1 serving = half cup)

Ingredients
- ¼ tsp. garlic powder
- 1 tsp. olive oil
- 1 tsp. onion powder
- ¼ cup chopped green bell pepper
- 1 cup firm tofu
- ⅛ tsp. turmeric
- ¼ cup chopped red bell pepper
- 1 minced clove garlic

Nutrition Per Serving

Calories	213 cal
Protein	18 g

Sodium	24 mg
Phosphorus	242 mg
Dietary Fiber	2 g
Potassium	467 mg

Directions

- Sauté the garlic and the two bell peppers in olive oil in a nonstick, medium-sized pan.
- Rinse the tofu and place it in the skillet. The remaining ingredients are added.
- Mix and cook till the tofu becomes a light golden brown, for approximately 20 minutes, on low to medium heat. Water from the mixture would evaporate.
- Serve the tofu

8. Southwest Baked Breakfast Egg Cups

12 Servings (1 serving = 2.5 oz. or 1 egg cup)

Ingredients

- 4 oz. shredded cheddar cheese
- 3 cups cooked rice
- 4 oz. diced green chilies
- ½ cup milk (skim)
- 2 oz. diced and drained pimentos
- ½ tsp. ground cumin
- 2 beaten eggs
- cooking spray (nonstick)
- ½ tsp. black pepper

Nutrition Per Serving

Calories	109 cal
Protein	5 g
Sodium	79 mg
Phosphorus	91 mg
Dietary Fiber	0.5 g
Potassium	82 mg

Directions

- Combine the rice, chilies, milk, 2 oz. of cheese, pimentos, cumin, eggs, and pepper in a big bowl.
- Use cooking spray, which is nonstick, to spray muffin cups.
- Spoon the mixture into 12 muffin cups equally. Sprinkle the remaining 2 oz. of cheese on top of each cup.

9. Mexican Tortilla And Egg Skillet Breakfast

6 Servings

Ingredients
- 2 sliced thin, green onions
- 8 eggs
- 1/4 cup ketchup (low salt)
- 1 tsp. chili powder
- 1 bag (6oz) broken up, unsalted tortilla chips
- 2 tbsp. Butter

Nutrition Per Serving

Calories	297 kcals
Protein	11 g
Sodium	267 mg
Phosphorus	179 mg
Dietary Fiber	2 g
Potassium	152 mg

Directions
- Beat the eggs until they are well mixed.
- Add the ketchup, onion, and chili powder. Beat it till it is well blended again. Then set aside.
- In a pan, melt the butter, add the sauté and tortilla chips until warmed through moderate heat. Stir in the mixture of eggs and scramble till the perfect consistency is reached. On heated plates, serve at once.

10. Fresh Fruit Compote

8 servings (serving size 1/2 cup)

Ingredients

- 1/4 cup frozen or fresh red raspberries (sweetened and not thawed)

- 1/2 cup frozen or fresh strawberries

- 1/2 cup pared, cut peaches.

- 1/2 cup frozen or fresh blackberries

- 1 Apple, diced into bite-size pieces

- 1/2 cup unsweetened, canned, or fresh orange juice

- 1/2 cup frozen or fresh blueberries

- 1 Banana, diced into bite-size pieces

Nutrition Per Serving

Calories	44 cal
Protein	0.5 g
Sodium	1 mg
Phosphorus	13 mg
Dietary Fiber	1.6 g
Potassium	140 mg

Directions
- Pour orange juice into a large bottle.
- Add all the mentioned ingredients.
- Gently toss.
- When utilizing frozen fruits, allow four hours at room temp to thaw.

11. Burritos with Mexican Sausage and Eggs

3 servings
Ingredients
- 3 beaten eggs
- 3 oz. of chorizo (Mexican sausage)
- 3 flour tortillas

Nutrition Per Serving

Calories	320 kcals
Protein	16 g
Sodium	659 mg
Phosphorus	170 mg
Dietary Fiber	1 g
Potassium	214 mg

Directions
- Fry the chorizo in a pan until the color is dark.
- Add the eggs and cook until its done.

- Fill hot tortillas with the mixture and roll-up. Cover the bottom side before rolling to prevent the filling from spilling out.

12. Orange Flavored Coffee

20 servings (serving size: 2 round tsp.)
Ingredients
- 3/4 cup sugar
- 1/2 cup coffee
- 1/2 tsp. orange peel, dried
- 1 cup Coffee-Mate Powder

Nutrition Per Serving

Calories	42 kcals
Protein	0.4 g
Sodium	4 mg
Phosphorus	14 mg
Dietary Fiber	0 g
Potassium	99 mg

Directions
- Blend the ingredients mentioned above in a blender until they are in powdered form.
- Add 2 round tsp. of the coffee mix in a cup with each serving. Then add boiling water and enjoy.

13. 40-Second Omelet

1 SERVING
Ingredients
- 2 tbsp. water
- 2 eggs
- 1/2 cup filling (meat, vegetables, seafood)
- 1 tbsp. unsalted butter

Nutrition Per Serving

Calories	255 cal
Protein	13 g
Sodium	145 mg
Phosphorus	195 mg
Dietary Fiber	2 g
Potassium	122 mg

Directions

- Whip the water and eggs together till they are blended.
- Heat butter in a 10-inch fry pan or omelet pan until just warm enough for a drop of water to sizzle.
- Pour the egg mixture onto it. The mixture should be placed on the edges instantly. Move cooked portions at the edges cautiously into the middle using an inverted pancake turner so that uncooked portions will touch the hot pan surface. Tilt the pan and move as needed.
- Continue until the egg is set and does not circulate. If required, fill the omelet with meat, 1/2 cup of vegetables, or seafood stuffing. If you are right-handed, place the filling on the left side, and if you are left-handed, on the right side.
- Fold the omelet in half using the pancake turner. Invert the omelet's bottom side facing up onto a tray.

14. Anytime Energy Bars

8 servings

Ingredients

- 1/2 tsp. ground cinnamon
- 1 cup rolled oats
- 3 tsp. chopped, unsalted peanuts
- 1/3 cup coconut, shredded
- 1/4 cup mini chocolate chips (semi-sweet)
- 3 eggs
- 3 tbsp. honey
- 1/3 cup applesauce

Nutrition Per Serving

Calories	206 cal
Protein	7 g
Sodium	35 mg
Phosphorus	163 mg
Dietary Fiber	8 g
Potassium	182 mg

Directions

- Heat the oven to 325° F. With cooking spray, grease a 9×9-inch plate.
- Combine the cinnamon, oats, chocolate chips, coconut, and peanuts in a large mixing dish.

- In a tiny mixing bowl, beat the eggs. Add honey, then applesauce, and combine properly.
- Add the mixture of eggs to the oat mixture and blend properly.
- Uniformly press the mixture into the bottom of the 9×9-inch greased plate.
- For 40 minutes, cook. Cool, and cut into bars.

15. Apple Bran Muffins

12 servings

Ingredients
- 1 1/2 cups wheat bran
- 2 cups wheat flour
- 1 1/4 tsp. baking soda
- 1 tbsp. grated orange rind
- 1/2 tsp. nutmeg
- 1 cup apple (chopped)
- 1/2 cup sunflower seeds or chopped nuts
- 1/2 cup raisins
- scant 2 cups sour milk or buttermilk
- 1 orange juice
- 1/2 cup molasses
- 1 beaten egg
- 2 tbsp. oil

Nutrition Per Serving

Calories	234 cal
Protein	7 g
Sodium	287 mg
Phosphorus	121 mg
Dietary Fiber	6 g
Potassium	446 mg

Directions
- Preheat the oven to 350°F.
- Stir together the bran, flour, nutmeg, and baking soda with a fork.
- Add the apples, orange rind, raisins, and seeds or nuts.
- To make two cups, drain 1 orange juice into a 2-cup measure, then add buttermilk.
- Combine the mixture of buttermilk with the molasses, egg, and oil, blend well.

- Stir the liquid ingredients with a few short strokes into the dry ingredients.
- Pour into oiled muffin tins, fill two-thirds of them thoroughly, then bake for at least 25 minutes.

16. Apple Filled Crepes

1 crepe serving

Ingredients
- 2 eggs (whole)
- 4 egg yolks
- 1 cup of flour
- 1/2 cup sugar
- 2 cups of milk
- 1/4 cup oil
- 1/2 cup brown sugar
- 4 apples
- 1/2 tsp. nutmeg
- 1/2 cup or 1 stick unsalted butter
- 1/2 tsp. cinnamon

Nutrition Per Serving

Calories	315 cal
Protein	5 g
Sodium	356 mg
Phosphorus	103 mg
Dietary Fiber	15 g
Potassium	160 mg

Directions
- Mix the egg yolks, sugar, whole eggs, oil, flour, and milk until the mixture is lump-free.
- Over medium heat, heat a tiny nonstick skillet.
- Use cooking spray to spray the pan.
- Using a 2 oz. ladle or 1/4 cup, add one scoop of batter into the pan, and then move the pan to scatter the crepe batter evenly on the bottom of the pan
- Cook for almost 20 seconds, and then turn the crepe by using a rubber spatula and again cook for about 10 seconds. Place aside the crepes as you render the filling.
- Peel, cut, and core the apples into 12 slices each.
- Heat the sauté pan.
- Then melt the butter and add the brown sugar.
- Toss in the cinnamon, apples, and nutmeg.

- Cook the apples till tender but not soggy. Allow them to cool.
- Assembling the Crepes: With around 2 tsp. of apple filling, fill the center of each crepe.
- Roll into a log.

17. Banana Oat Shake

2 servings

Ingredients
- 2/3 cup skim milk
- 1/2 cup chilled, cooked oatmeal
- 1 tbsp. wheat germ
- 2 tbsp. brown sugar
- 1/2 banana (frozen), cut into chunks
- 1 1/2 tsp. vanilla extract

Nutrition Per Serving

Calories	172 cal
Protein	6 g
Sodium	42 mg
Phosphorus	160 mg
Potassium	297 mg

Directions
- In a blender, put the oatmeal and blend for a few minutes.
- Add the brown sugar, milk, vanilla, wheat germ, and 1/2 banana. Blend them until smooth and thick.
- If needed, serve with ice.

18. Banana-Apple Smoothie

1 serving

Ingredients
- 1/2 cup yogurt, plain
- 1/2 peeled banana, cut into chunks
- 1/4 cup skim milk
- 1/2 cup applesauce, unsweetened
- 2 tbsp. oat bran
- 1 tbsp. honey

Nutrition Per Serving

Calories	292 cal

Protein	9 g
Sodium	103 mg
Phosphorus	140 mg
Potassium	609 mg

Directions
- In a blender, put the banana, milk, yogurt, honey, and applesauce.
- Blend until perfectly smooth.
- Add the oat bran and mix until it is thickened.

19. Berrylicious Smoothie

2 servings

Ingredients
- 2/3 cup firm silken tofu
- 1/4 cup juice cocktail of cranberry
- 1/2 cup unsweetened, frozen blueberries
- 1/2 cup unsweetened, frozen raspberries
- 1/2 tsp. powdered lemonade
- 1 tsp. vanilla extract

Nutrition Per Serving

Calories	115 cal
Protein	6 g
Sodium	14 mg
Phosphorus	80 mg
Dietary Fiber	1 g
Potassium	223 mg

Directions
- In a blender, pour juice.
- Add the remaining ingredients.
- Mix until thoroughly smooth.
- Serve instantly and enjoy!

20. Biscuits with Master Mix

12 servings

Ingredients
- 2/3 cup Water
- 3 cups Master Mix

Nutrition Per Serving

Calories	174 cal
Protein	3 g
Sodium	171 mg
Phosphorus	51 mg
Dietary Fiber	10 g
Potassium	81 mg

Directions
- Preheat the oven to 450°F.
- Mix the ingredients and blend properly.
- Let them stand 5 minutes.
- Knead the dough approximately 15 times on a lightly floured board.
- Roll out to half-inch thickness and slice till you've 12 biscuits using a flour cutter.
- Put them on a non-greased baking sheet 2 inches apart.
- Bake until golden brown, for 10-12 minutes.

21. Bran Breakfast Bars

12 servings

Ingredients
- 1/3 cup med. dates or chopped raisins, diced
- 1 cup boiling water
- 1/2 cup wheat flour
- 1 cup oatmeal
- 1 1/2 cups bran
- 1/3 cup oil (soybean, safflower, or corn)
- 3 tbsp. the brown-type sugar substitute, granular

Nutrition Per Serving

Calories	158 cal
Protein	4 g
Sodium	2 mg
Phosphorus	142 mg
Potassium	148 mg

Directions
- Fill the diced fruit with hot water.
- Leave it to stand for 20 minutes at least.
- In a big mixing bowl, combine the dried ingredients.
- Drain fruit. To make 1 cup, add hot water to the drained liquid and place it in a blender with the oil.

- For 1 minute, blend.
- Pour in the dry ingredients instantly and combine properly.
- Add remix and fruit.
- Layer the batter in an 8"x10" nonstick baking dish.
- Level with your fingertips or spatula and then mark the cuttings: four narrow rows and broad six rows.
- Bake for 22 minutes in a preheated oven at 375F.
- Cool on a shelf.
- If storing for longer than 2 days, refrigerate or freeze.

22. Burritos Rapidos

4 servings

Ingredients
- 1 1/2 tsp. olive oil or canola oil
- 1/2 of diced red bell pepper
- 4 green, sliced thin onions (scallions)
- 8 beaten eggs
- 4 (6-inch) corn tortillas

Nutrition Per Serving

Calories	232 cal
Protein	14 g
Sodium	152 mg
Phosphorus	207 mg
Dietary Fiber	6 g
Potassium	211 mg

Directions
- Heat oil over low heat in a medium frying pan.
- Add the green onion and bell pepper and cook for around 3 minutes, until softened.
- Add the eggs and scramble for 5 minutes or until the eggs are thoroughly cooked.
- Place the tortillas between 2 damp paper towels and place them on a dish.
- Place the tortillas in the microwave for around 2 minutes.
- Spoon the mixture of eggs into warm tortillas.
- Roll up to eat the tortillas.
- Try sprinkling chili powder or applying a splash of hot sauce for a little kick.

23. Fresh Fruit Lassi

2 servings

Ingredients
- 1/2 cup milk
- 1 cup yogurt, plain
- 1-3 tbsp. sugar to taste
- 1/2 cup mango juice (or apricot or peach nectar)
- 1/2 tsp. rose water (optional)
- 1/4 tsp. cardamon (optional)
- 1/4 cup lime juice (optional)

Nutrition Per Serving

Calories	169 cal
Protein	9 g
Sodium	143 mg
Phosphorus	59 mg
Dietary Fiber	2 g
Potassium	98 mg

Directions
- Put all the ingredients in a food processor or blender and mix for 2 minutes, then pour and serve in individual glasses.

24. Fruit Bars

24 servings

Ingredients
- 1/2 cup sugar
- 1 tsp. baking powder
- 2 cups flour
- 1/2 cup vegetable oil
- 1/4 cup water
- 1 egg
- 1 cup jam (grape, strawberry, blackberry, raspberry)
- 1 tsp. vanilla extract

Nutrition Per Serving

Calories	131 cal

Protein	1 g
Sodium	24 mg
Phosphorus	120 mg
Potassium	14 mg

Directions
- Preheat the oven to 400°F.
- Mix the sugar, flour, and baking powder together.
- Stir the oil till crumbly.
- Add the vanilla extract, water, and egg and blend properly
- In an 8×8 or 9×9-inch greased pan, place 2/3 of the batter.
- Distribute uniformly with jam
- To make crumbs on top, use the leftover batter.
- For 25-30 mins, bake.
- Cool in a pan then cut into 24 bars.

Chapter 3: Lunch Ideas for Dialysis Diets

Have a look at our collection of burgers, salads, and other delicious ideas for lunch. You can also toss a salad and throw in a hard-boiled egg, just go simple on the pre-made salad dressing, which can be a hidden phosphorus source. Better yet, with vinegar or lemon and oil, make your own.

1. Lemon Orzo Spring Salad

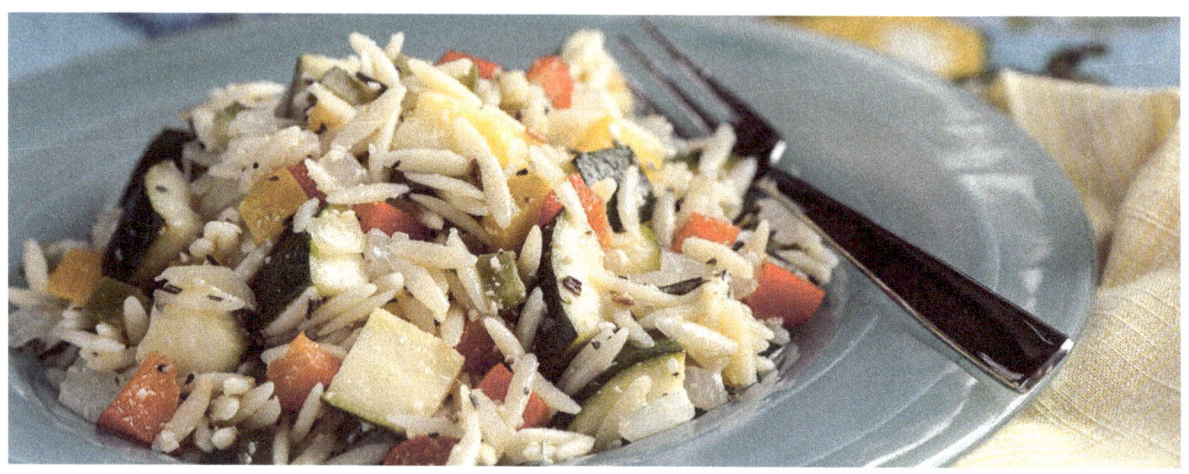

4 servings (1 serving = 1 ½ cup portion)

Ingredients
- ¼ cup fresh, diced yellow peppers
- ¼ box or ¾ cup orzo pasta
- 1 tsp. lemon zest
- ¼ cup fresh, diced green peppers
- 2 cups medium-cubed, fresh zucchini
- ¼ cup fresh, diced red peppers
- 2 tbsp. chopped fresh rosemary
- 3 tbsp. fresh lemon juice
- ½ tsp. dried oregano
- ½ cup fresh, diced Vidalia or red onion
- ¼ cup and 2 tbsp. olive oil
- ½ tsp. black pepper
- 3 tbsp. Parmesan cheese, grated
- ½ tsp. red pepper flakes

Nutrition Per Serving

Calories	330 cal
Protein	6 g
Sodium	79 mg
Phosphorus	134 mg

| Dietary Fiber | 5 g |
| Potassium | 376 mg |

Directions
- Cook the orzo pasta, drain, and let sit according to the package instructions. (Not to rinse.)
- On moderate heat, sauté the onions, zucchini, and peppers with 2 tbsp. of oil in a large mixing pan until translucent.
- In a big bowl, add the lemon zest, lemon juice, half a cup of olive oil, rosemary, cheese, oregano, pepper, and red pepper flakes.
- In a big bowl, add the orzo pasta and sautéed vegetables and fold gently till it's mixed.
- Serve

2. Shrimp Noodle and Chilled Veggie Salad

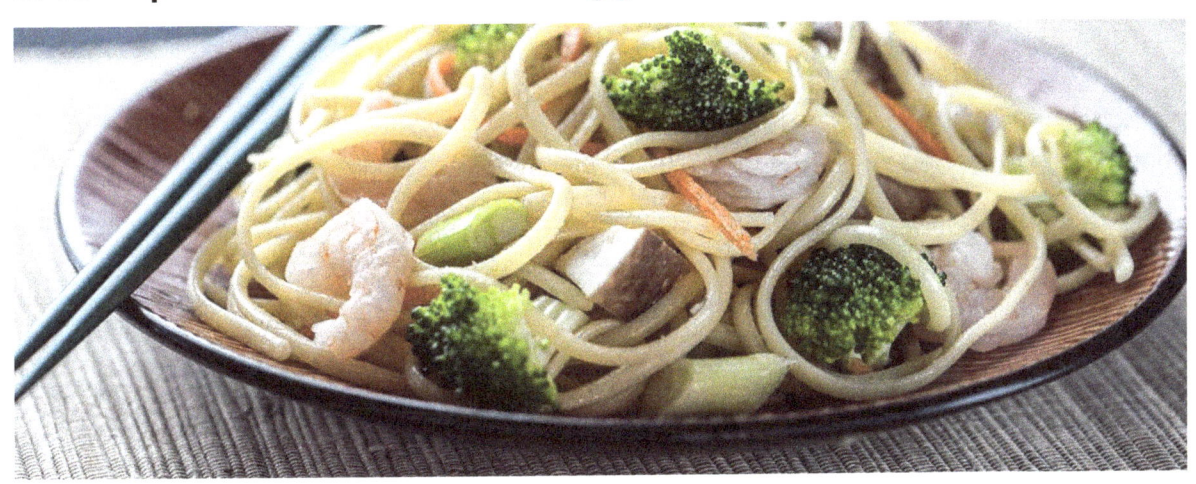

10 serving (1 serving = 1 3/4 cup)

Ingredients
- 4 cups cooked, deveined, peeled, tailless, and cut in half cocktail shrimp; or 14-oz. pack of salad shrimp, cooked
- 1 lb. package of dry Spaghetti, chilled and cooked noodles (do not rinse)
- 2 cups broccoli florets (fresh)
- 1 cup scallions (fresh), sliced on the bias
- 2 cups fresh, chopped shitake mushrooms
- 2 tbsp. sesame oil
- 1 cup shredded, fresh carrots
- ½ cup rice wine vinegar
- 2 tsp. chili oil
- 1 tbsp. chopped, fresh ginger
- 2 tbsp. chopped, fresh garlic
- ¼ cup lime juice (2 limes), and zest of 1 lime (1 tbsp.)

- ¼ cup soy sauce substitute (low-sodium)

Low-Sodium Soy Sauce Substitute (1 cup):
- 1 tsp. low-sodium soy sauce
- 4 tsp. low sodium Better Than Bouillon Chicken Base
- 2 tsp. dark molasses
- 4 tsp. Balsamic vinegar
- ¼ tsp. white pepper
- ¼ tsp. ground ginger
- 1½ cups water
- ¼ tsp. garlic powder

Nutrition Per Serving

Calories	254 cal
Protein	13 g
Sodium	433 mg
Phosphorus	229 mg
Dietary Fiber	3 g
Potassium	325 mg

Directions
- Combine the substitute soy sauce ingredients in a small saucepan.
- On medium flame, stir. Allow it to slightly thicken and reduce to around 1 cup. Store the rest in the fridge.
- Then, in a big bowl, combine the ingredients together and set aside.
- Blend together the remaining ingredients in the blender until well mixed, around 1 minute.
- Pour the dressing mixture over the pasta mixture. Toss till it's covered well, then eat.

3. Chicken Broccoli Stromboli

4 servings (1 serving = ¼ of Stromboli)
Ingredients
- 2 cups fresh, blanched broccoli florets
- 1 lb. pizza dough
- 1 cup low-salt, shredded mozzarella cheese
- 2 cups cooked chicken breast, diced
- 1 tbsp. chopped fresh oregano
- 1 tbsp. chopped fresh garlic
- 2 tbsp. flour
- 1 tsp. red pepper flakes, crushed
- 2 tbsp. olive oil

Nutrition Per Serving

Calories	522 cal
Protein	38 g
Sodium	607 mg
Phosphorus	400 mg
Dietary Fiber	2.9 g
Potassium	546 mg

Directions

- Preheat the oven to 400° F.
- In a big bowl, mix the chicken, pepper flakes, cheese, garlic, oregano, broccoli and set aside.
- Powder tabletop with flour and roll dough out until you hit a rectangular form of 11" x 14".
- Place the chicken mixture along the longest line, about two inches from the side of the dough.
- Pinch and roll the seam and ends till sealed tightly.
- Use olive oil to brush the top and make 3 tiny slits on the surface of the dough.
- Bake on the lightly greased baking sheet tray for 8-12 minutes or till golden brown.
- Remove, give 3-5 minutes to settle, then slice and serve.

4. Crispy and Cool Cucumber Salad

4 servings (1 serving = ½ cup)

Ingredients

- 2 tbsp. Caesar or Italian salad dressing
- 2 cups fresh cucumber, sliced into ¼-inch slices (peeling is optional)
- Ground black pepper (according to taste)

Nutrition Per Serving

Calories	27 cal
Protein	0 g
Sodium	74 mg
Phosphorus	14 mg
Dietary Fiber	0 g
Potassium	90 mg

Directions

- Combine the salad dressing and cucumber in a medium-size bowl with a lid.
- Shake to coat after covering with a lid
- Use ground black pepper to sprinkle. Refrigerate.
- Serve

5. Savory and Smoky Salmon Dip

12 servings (1 serving = ¼ cup)
Ingredients
- 1 lb. fresh boneless, skinless salmon (cut into 4 pieces)
- 2 tsp. smoked paprika
- 1 cup cream cheese
- ¼ cup capers
- Zest of half a lemon (1 tsp.) and ¼ cup lemon juice
- 2 tsp. finely diced, red onions
- 1 tsp. ground black pepper
- 1 tbsp. chopped, fresh parsley

Nutrition Per Serving

Calories	133 cal
Protein	10 g
Sodium	147 mg
Phosphorus	110 mg
Dietary Fiber	0 mg
Potassium	259 mg

Directions
- For 4-6 minutes on medium-high heat, scoop up the salmon in two cups of water and 1 tsp. of smoked paprika; the pot must be closed but should not hit a boil. Remove and chill for around 30 minutes
- Mix together all of the other ingredients till smooth. Split the salmon into bite-sized bits and fold them into a mixture of cream cheese.
- Chill for 20-30 minutes, the salmon dip. Serve with carrots, celery sticks, corn chips or wrapped in an iceberg lettuce leaf.

6. Herb-Roasted Chicken Breasts

4 servings (1 serving = 4 oz.)
Ingredients
- 1 medium onion
- 1 lb. skinless, boneless chicken breasts
- 2 tbsp. herb and garlic seasoning blend
- 1–2 garlic cloves
- ¼ cup olive oil
- 1 tsp. ground black pepper

Nutrition Per Serving

Calories	270 cal
Protein	26 g
Sodium	53 mg
Phosphorus	252 mg
Dietary Fiber	0.6 g
Potassium	491 mg

Directions

Marinating:
- Chop the garlic and onion and put them in a dish. Add seasoning, olive oil and ground pepper.
- To marinade, add chicken breasts, cover, and refrigerate overnight or at least 4 hours.

Baking:
- Preheat the oven to 350°F.
- Line a baking sheet with foil and put the chicken breasts on the pan
- Pour the rest of the marinade over the chicken breasts and bake for 20 minutes at 350 ° F.
- Broil for an estimated 5 minutes until brown.

7. Fired-Up Zucchini Burger

4 servings (1 serving = 1 burger)

Ingredients
- 1 cup shredded zucchini
- 1 lb. ground turkey meat
- 1 minced and seeded jalapeño pepper (sliced lengthwise)
- ½ cup minced onion
- 1 tsp. Extra Spicy Blend
- 1 egg
- 1 tsp. mustard (optional)
- 2 fresh, seeded poblano peppers (sliced in half lengthwise)

Nutrition Per Serving

Calories	211 cal
Protein	25 g
Sodium	128 mg
Phosphorus	280 mg
Dietary Fiber	1.6 g
Potassium	475 mg

Directions

- Thoroughly mix the ingredients. Create 4 turkey burger patties of meat mixture. Turkey burgers can be grilled on a barbecue or an electronic griddle. When the skin is blistered and tender, the peppers could be grilled with turkey burgers. At a 165°F temperature or until the middle is no longer pink barbecue turkey burgers.
- Serve on a hamburger bun, top the patty with diced grilled pepper and eat.

8. Egg Fried Rice

10 servings (1 serving = ½ cup)

Ingredients

- 2 eggs
- 2 tsp. dark sesame oil
- 1 tbsp. canola oil
- 2 egg whites
- ⅓ cup chopped green onions
- ¼ tsp. ground black pepper
- 1 cup bean sprouts
- 1 cup thawed frozen peas
- 4 cups cold cooked rice

Nutrition Per Serving

Calories	137 cal
Protein	5 g
Sodium	38 mg
Phosphorus	67 mg
Dietary Fiber	1.3 g
Potassium	89 mg

Directions

- In a tiny bowl, mix the eggs, sesame oil, and egg whites together. Stir thoroughly and set aside.
- Heat canola oil over medium to high heat in a broad nonstick skillet.
- Add the mixture of eggs and stir-fry until ready.
- Add the green onions and bean sprouts. For 2 minutes, stir-fry.
- Have peas and rice included. Continue to stir-fry until fully heated.
- Use black pepper for spice and serve immediately.

9. Pea Salad and Ginger-Lime Vinaigrette

6 servings (1 serving = ½ cup)

Ingredients
- 1 cup thawed or fresh frozen sweet peas
- 1 cup snow peas
- 1 cup sugar snap peas

Vinaigrette:
- ¼ cup lime juice, fresh
- 1 tsp. reduced-sodium soy sauce
- 2 tsp. chopped, fresh ginger
- 1 tbsp. sesame seeds
- 1 tsp. fresh lime zest
- 1 tbsp. hot sesame oil
- ½ cup canola oil

Nutrition Per Serving

Calories	225 cal
Protein	3 g
Sodium	70 mg
Phosphorus	40 mg
Dietary Fiber	1.8 g
Potassium	117 mg

Directions
- In a hot skillet, gently toast the sesame seeds, flipping them continuously for around 3-5 minutes.
- Blanch all 3 forms of peas for 2 minutes in a big pot of boiling water on high heat, rinse and shake them in a cool water bowl. Switch to a strainer and thoroughly drain.
- Whisk the black pepper, soy sauce, zest, and lime juice in a small bowl until well-mixed, around 1-2 minutes.
- Continue whisking, with the ginger added. Drizzle in the grapeseed or canola oil gently, then add the sesame oil and blend until well mixed.
- Combine the pea mixture and salad dressing in a large bowl. Place the sesame seeds and black pepper to taste and serve.

10. Veggie Vindaloo with Naan

6 servings (1 serving = 1 mini naan bread)

Ingredients
- 2 diced shallots
- 2 tbsp. ghee oil, canola oil, or mustard oil
- ¼ cup diced zucchini

- ¼ cup diced and peeled eggplant
- ½ cup mixed, diced green and red peppers
- ¼ cup cauliflower
- 2 tbsp. fresh lime juice
- 1 cup cooked quinoa
- ½ cup queso fresco or paneer
- 4–6 mini naan bread
- 2 tbsp. chopped fresh cilantro

Seasoning mix:
- ½ tsp. turmeric
- 2 tsp. curry powder
- ¼ tsp. ground ginger
- ½ tsp. ground red chili pepper flakes
- ½ tsp. ground cumin
- ¼ tsp. ground cloves
- ¼ tsp. ground cinnamon

Nutrition Per Serving

Calories	306 cal
Protein	11 g
Sodium	403 mg
Phosphorus	238 mg
Dietary Fiber	4.7 g
Potassium	238 mg

Directions
- Heat the oil to medium-high in a broad sauté pan, then add the eggplant, shallots, cauliflower, mixed peppers, and zucchini and sauté for 2-4 minutes. Slightly translucent and yet crunchy, the vegetables should be. Add a mixture of seasoning and whisk until well-mixed.
- Mix in the lime juice, cooked quinoa, cheese, and cilantro and switch off the heat.
- Serve whether cold or hot.
- To serve chilled: Chill filling. Add equally to the naan bread
- To serve hot: Randomly spread the veggie mix on top of the hot naan bread.

11. Jalapeño-Lime Burger and Smoked Mozzarella

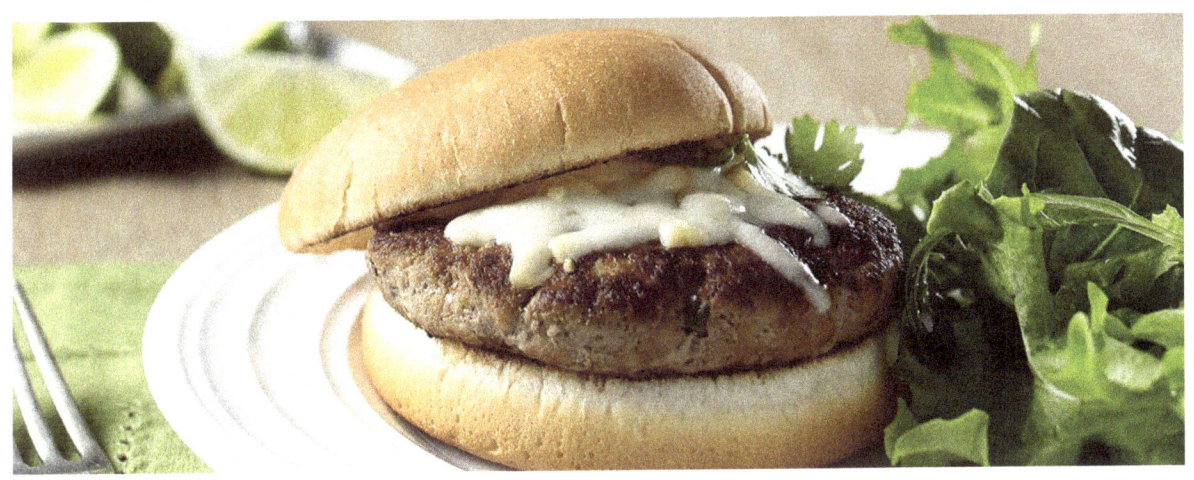

8 servings (1 serving = 1 burger)

Ingredients
- zest of 1 lime and juice of 2 limes
- 2 tbsp. diced jalapeño
- 1 tbsp. Worcestershire sauce (reduced sodium)
- 1 tbsp. ground black pepper, fresh
- 8 slices of mozzarella cheese and skim milk
- 4 tbsp. olive oil
- 8 toasted hamburger buns
- 2 lb. ground turkey

Nutrition Per Serving

Calories	407 cal
Protein	32 g
Sodium	435 mg
Phosphorus	399 mg
Dietary Fiber	0.9 g
Potassium	378 mg

Directions
- Combine the ingredients plus 2 tsp. of olive oil in a medium-size bowl. Shape 8 turkey burger patties of similar size and brush them gently with 2 tsp. of olive oil.
- Heat half of the canola oil to medium-high in a large nonstick sauté pan over medium-high heat.
- Cook the burgers for 5-7 minutes on each side, turning once or until an instant-read thermometer hits an internal temperature of 165° F.
- Add about 2 tbsp. of cheese to each burger and melt in an oven set or toaster oven to broil.
- Serve on a toasted bun for each turkey burger.

12. Crunchy Quinoa Salad

8 servings (1 serving = ½ cup)

Ingredients

- 1 cup quinoa (rinsed)
- 2 cups of water
- 5 diced cherry tomatoes
- ¼ cup grated parmesan cheese
- ½ cup diced and seeded cucumbers
- 3 chopped green onions
- ¼ cup chopped, fresh mint
- 4 tbsp. olive oil
- ½ cup chopped, flat-leaf parsley
- 2 tbsp. fresh lemon juice
- 1 tbsp. grated lemon rind, zest
- ½ head Bibb or Boston lettuce (separated into cups)

Nutrition Per Serving

Calories	158 cal
Protein	5 g
Sodium	46 mg
Phosphorus	129 mg
Dietary Fiber	2.3 g
Potassium	237 mg

Directions

- Rinse the quinoa once clear under cool running water and rinse it properly.
- Over medium-high heat, put the quinoa in a pan and toast for 2 minutes, mixing periodically. Mix in 2 cups of water and get it to a boil. Decrease the heat to low, then cover the pan and cook for 8-10 minutes. Let it cook and fluff it with a fork.
- Combine the lemon juice, herbs, olive oil, and zest with the onions, tomatoes, and cucumbers. To the mixture, add the cooled quinoa.
- Spoon the mixture into cups of lettuce, then dust the top with parmesan cheese.

13. Low Salt Macaroni with Cheese

4 servings

Ingredients

- 2 to 3 cups of boiling water

- 2 cups noodles

- 1 tsp. salt-free butter or margarine

- 1/2 cup cheddar cheese, grated.

- 1/4 tsp. mustard, dried

Nutrition Per Serving

Calories	163 kcals
Protein	6 g
Sodium	114 mg
Phosphorus	138 mg
Dietary Fiber	3 g
Potassium	39 mg

Directions
- Boil the water, add the noodles, and cook until soft, around 5-7 minutes.
- Drain.
- Sprinkle with cheese, whisk in mustard and butter while it's still really hot.
- (Optional: Bake for 10 to 15 minutes at 350 or until the surface is golden brown for a tastier crunch.)

14. Chicken Fusilli Salad

4 servings
Ingredients
Dressing

- 1/4 cup vinegar

- 1/2 cup olive oil

- 1/4 tsp. Basil

- 1 tsp. sugar

- 1/2 tsp. white pepper

Salad

- 8 oz. cold, diced cooked chicken
- 3 cups fusilli pasta, cooked
- 1/2 cup red pepper, chopped
- 1/2 cup defrosted frozen peas
- 1 medium carrot (sliced thinly)
- 2 cups lettuce, shredded
- 1 cup zucchini, sliced

Nutrition Per Serving

Calories	477 kcals
Protein	18 g
Sodium	65 mg
Phosphorus	239 mg
Dietary Fiber	8 g
Potassium	446 mg

Directions
- Place the dressing ingredients in the jar, cover it with a lid and shake well to combine the ingredients together. Chill for 2 hours at least. Before mixing with the salad, shake again.
- In a big dish, combine the pasta, peas, chicken, zucchini, carrot and red pepper together.
- Add some dressing and toss well. On 4 dishes, divide the lettuce and top with the salad mixture.

15. Italian Eggplant Salad

4 servings

Ingredients

- 1 small, chopped onion
- 1 medium, chopped tomato
- 3 cups eggplant, cubed
- 1 clove, chopped garlic
- 2 tbsp. white wine vinegar
- 1/4 tsp. black pepper
- 1/2 tsp. oregano
- 3 tbsp. olive oil

Nutrition Per Serving

Calories	69 kcals
Protein	1 g
Sodium	2 mg
Phosphorus	15 mg
Potassium	118 mg

Directions
- In a saucepan, add the eggplants to the boiling water.
- Reheat to boiling, heat reduction.
- Cover and simmer for around 10 minutes, until tender; rinse.
- Place the onions and eggplant in a glass dish.
- Mix the garlic, pepper, and vinegar together.
- Pour over the onions and eggplant, toss.
- Just before serving, stir in the oil.

16. Chicken Waldorf Salad

4 servings (serving size: 3/4 cup)

Ingredients
- 8 oz. cubed and cooked chicken or turkey
- 1/2 cup chopped apple
- 1/2 cup chopped celery
- 2 tbsp. raisins

- 1/2 tbsp. ground ginger
- 1/2 cup Miracle Whip

Nutrition Per Serving

Calories	224 kcals
Protein	14 g
Sodium	233 mg
Phosphorus	129 mg
Dietary Fiber	0.7 g
Potassium	234 mg

Directions

- Mix the ingredients till well blended.
- If it will remain in the refrigerator for a while to mix flavors, it is best.

17. Chicken and Bow-Tie Pasta

6 servings

Ingredients

- 8 oz. chicken breast
- 3 cups bow-tie pasta, cooked
- 1/4 cup olive oil
- 2 cloves garlic
- 1/2 cup green onions, chopped
- 1-1/2 cups frozen, chopped broccoli
- 1 tsp. ground basil
- 1 cup red pepper, chopped
- 1 cup reduced-sodium chicken broth or homemade without salt
- 3/4 cup white wine
- 1/4 tsp. cayenne pepper

Nutrition Per Serving

Calories	258 kcals
Protein	13 g
Sodium	50 mg
Phosphorus	173 mg
Dietary Fiber	5 g
Potassium	338 mg

Directions
- Sauté the garlic in a large skillet with oil.
- Add the chicken breast, slice into tiny strips and brown.
- Add the remaining ingredients and allow for 15 minutes to simmer.
- Mix and serve promptly with cooked bow-tie pasta.

18. Burritos Rapidos, Fajtas

4 servings

Ingredients
- 1/2 cup green or red pepper, diced
- 4 Corn tortillas
- 2 eggs or leftover fish, chicken, or meat
- 1/2 cup white or green onion, diced

Toppings:
- cheddar cheese (grated), lettuce, sour cream, and fresh salsa

Nutrition Per Serving

Calories	93 kcals
Protein	8 g
Sodium	59 mg
Phosphorus	139 mg
Dietary Fiber	2 g
Potassium	177 mg

Directions
- Spray the frypan with a nonstick spray. Add the onion and peppers and cook till the onion is translucent and the color of the peppers is bright.
- Add the meat or eggs and simmer until done, stirring occasionally.
- Meanwhile, cover the corn tortillas in a wet paper towel and microwave for around 1 minute.
- With toppings, serve.

19. Apple Rice Salad

4 SERVINGS

Ingredients
- 1 tbsp. olive oil
- 2 tbsp. balsamic vinegar
- 2 tsp. Dijon or brown mustard
- 2 tsp. honey
- 1/4 tsp. garlic powder
- 1 tbsp. finely shredded orange peel
- 2 cups chopped apples (about 2 medium)
- 2 cups cooked rice (chilled)
- 2 tbsp. shelled, unsalted sunflower seeds
- 1 cup thinly sliced celery

Nutrition Per Serving

Calories	238 cal
Protein	4 g
Sodium	227 mg
Phosphorus	82 mg
Dietary Fiber	3 g
Potassium	238 mg

Directions
- Stir together the olive oil, vinegar, mustard, honey, garlic powder, and orange peel in a small bowl. Mix thoroughly and put aside.
- Combine the apples, rice, sunflower seeds, and celery in a large bowl. Toss once blended well.
- Drizzle over the dressing on the rice salad mixture and mix till the salad is well seasoned.
- Serve instantly or cover for up to 24 hours and refrigerate.

20. Beef Barley Soup

10 SERVINGS

Ingredients
- 2 pounds beef stew meat (diced 1-inch cubes)
- 1/2 tsp. black pepper
- 1 cup onion, chopped
- 1/4 cup vegetable oil (divided)
- 2 diced carrots
- 1/2 cup mushrooms, sliced

- 1/4 tsp. dried thyme
- 1/2 tsp. minced garlic
- 3 cups of water
- 1/2 cup barley
- 1 can (14.5 oz.) low sodium chicken broth
- 2 diced and soaked potatoes
- 1 frozen package (16 oz.) of vegetables

Nutrition Per Serving

Calories	270 cal
Protein	23 g
Sodium	105 mg
Phosphorus	250 mg
Dietary Fiber	10 g
Potassium	678 mg

Directions
- Beef with pepper seasoning.
- In a stew pot, add 2 tsp. of oil and sauté for 5 minutes.
- Add 2 more tsp. of oil and add some mushrooms, onions and carrots.
- Sauté and stir often for 5 minutes.
- Add the thyme and garlic and sauté for 3 minutes.
- Add the water and chicken broth to the pot.
- Add the mixed barley, potatoes, and vegetables.
- Mix and bring it to a boil.
- Cover and minimize heat.
- Simmer for 1 to 1 and a half hours.

21. Canned Fish Tacos

2 servings

Ingredients
- 2 tsp. oil
- 2 tbsp. chopped onion
- 1/2 cup frozen or canned corn
- 1 can rinsed and drained tuna
- 1/2 tsp. chili powder
- 1/4 cup diced, canned tomatoes (no salt added)
- 4 corn tortillas

Nutrition Per Serving

Calories	215.8 cal
Protein	12 g
Sodium	477 mg
Phosphorus	5.7 mg
Dietary Fiber	1.5 g
Potassium	121 mg

Directions
- Cook the onions in the oil on medium heat in a frying pan before they become clear.
- Add the corn, tuna, chili powder, and tomatoes.
- Cook until thoroughly heated, for 3-5 minutes.
- Serve with tortillas that are warm. Add, if needed, lettuce, sour cream, and hot sauce.
- For canned chicken or salmon, you may substitute canned tuna. Instead of fresh onion, consider using 1/2 tsp. onion powder.

22. Chicken and Orange Salad Sandwich

6 servings

Ingredients
- 1/2 cup diced celery
- 1 cup cooked chicken, chopped
- 1/4 cup finely sliced onion
- 1/2 cup chopped green pepper
- 1/3 cup mayonnaise
- 1 cup Mandarin oranges

Nutrition Per Serving

Calories	162 cal
Protein	12 g
Sodium	93 mg
Phosphorus	106 mg
Potassium	241 mg

Directions
- Mix together the celery, chicken, onion, and green pepper.
- Add mayonnaise and mandarin oranges.
- Gently mix.
- Serve on bread.

23. Cowboy Caviar Bean with Rice Salad

6 servings

Ingredients
- 3 cups cooked rice
- 1/2 cup cooked, frozen or fresh corn
- 1/2 cup canola oil or olive oil
- 1/4 cup lime juice
- 1 tbsp. Dijon mustard
- 2 tbsp. brown sugar
- 1/2 cup diced red bell pepper
- 1/2 cup chopped cilantro
- 1/2 tsp. black pepper
- 1 seeded and diced jalapeño
- 1/2 cup rinsed and drained, low sodium black beans, canned

Nutrition Per Serving

Calories	237 cal
Protein	4 g
Sodium	101 mg
Phosphorus	40 mg
Potassium	195 mg

Directions
- Prepare the corn and rice and let it cool.
- Whisk together the lime juice, brown sugar, oil, black pepper, and mustard to form the dressing.
- Combine all the other ingredients in a big bowl.
- Pour the dressing over the salad and Mix.
- Chill in the refrigerator for 1 hour.

24. Curry Chicken Salad

8 servings

Ingredients
- 1/2 cup raisins
- 1 tsp. curry powder
- 3/4 cup or 1 1/2 cups each light sour cream or mayonnaise
- 2 cups chicken or turkey, cooked
- 1/2 cup reduced-sodium Mango Chutney (such as Major Grey)
- 3 chopped celery stalks
- 1/2 cup nuts (hazelnuts, cashews, sliced almonds, or pecans)
- 4 chopped green onions

Nutrition Per Serving

Calories	304 cal

Protein	21 g
Sodium	231 mg
Phosphorus	65 mg
Potassium	361 mg

Directions

- For the dressing, mix curry powder, chutney, and mayo together.
- Toss the green onions, chicken, nuts, celery, and raisins in a bowl, then combine the dressing with the mixture.
- Allow the refrigerator to cool overnight for more flavor.

Chapter 4: Dinner Ideas for Dialysis Diets

1. Pesto-Crusted Catfish

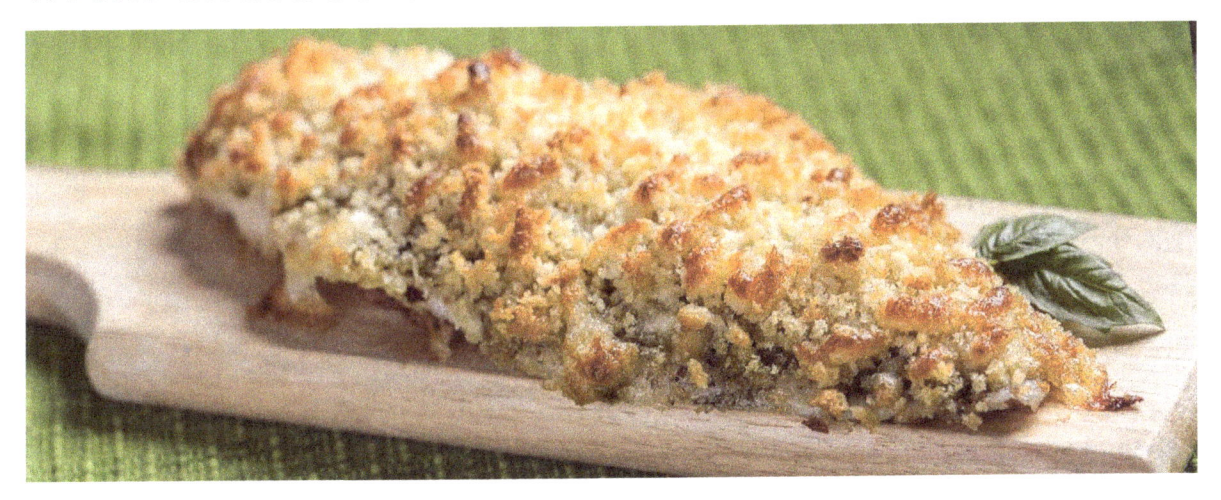

6 servings (1 serving = 5-oz. portion)

Ingredients
- 4 tsp. pesto
- 2 tbsp. olive oil
- 2 lb. catfish (filleted and boned), 6 5-oz. pieces
- ½ cup mozzarella cheese
- ¾ cup breadcrumbs, panko

Chef McCargo's Seasoning Blend:
- 1 tsp. onion powder
- ½ tsp. red pepper flakes
- ½ tsp. dried oregano
- 1 tsp. garlic powder
- ½ tsp. black pepper

Nutrition Per Serving

Calories	321 cal
Protein	26 g
Sodium	272 mg
Phosphorus	417 mg
Dietary Fiber	0.8 g
Potassium	576 mg

Directions
- Preheat the oven to 400° F.

- In a small cup, combine all the seasonings and start to sprinkle even quantities on both sides of the fish.
- Spread similar quantities of pesto on the top of the fillets (1 tsp. each) and set them aside.
- Mix the cheese, breadcrumbs, and oil in a medium bowl and dredge the fish's pesto side in the mixture until well covered.
- Liberally spray or grease baking sheet tray with oil and place fish pesto on the sheet tray side while leaving space among fillets.
- Bake on the bottom rack for 15-20 minutes at 400 ° F till required brownness.
- After cooking, leave to rest for 10 minutes and remove from the tray to avoid breaking the fish.

2. Smokin' Chicken and Mustard Sauce

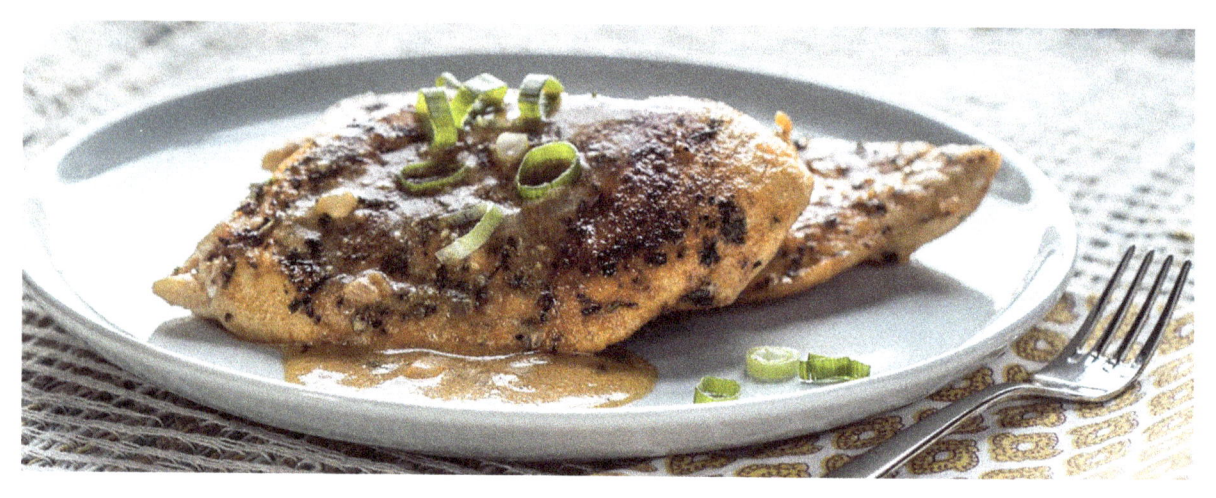

8 servings (1 serving = 4-oz. portion)

Ingredients
- ¼ cup shallots, diced
- 2 lb. chicken breast, thinly sliced (or skinless, boneless chicken breast, thin)
- ½ cup flour
- ¼ cup fresh chopped scallions
- ½ cubed and chilled, stick unsalted butter
- 2 cups chicken stock, low-sodium
- ½ cup canola oil
- 2 tbsp. brown mustard
- 1 tbsp. low sodium Better Than Bouillon' Chicken Base.'

Seasonings:
- ½ tsp. Italian seasoning
- ½ tsp. black pepper
- 1 tbsp. smoked paprika

- 1 tbsp. dried parsley

Nutrition Per Serving

Calories	361 cal
Protein	28 g
Sodium	300 mg
Phosphorus	278 mg
Dietary Fiber	0.6 g
Potassium	471 mg

Directions
- In a tiny bowl, blend the Italian seasoning, pepper, parsley and paprika together.
- Sprinkle half of it on the breast of the chicken and apply the rest to the flour.
- Heat the oil over medium-high heat in a large skillet.
- Remove and set aside 3 tbsp. of seasoned flour
- Dredge the chicken in the remaining flour and sauté on each side for 2 to 3 minutes.
- Remove the chicken and put it aside to rest on a tray. Add sauté and shallots until mildly translucent; extract all but a few tbsp. of oil.
- Mix until smooth in the flour and continue to add stock steadily while continuing to whisk. Lower the heat and whisk in mustard, unsalted butter, and chicken bouillon after 5 minutes of cooking over medium-high heat.
- Turn the heat off and return the chicken and all the juice drippings back to the pan from the plate and stir. Garnish and plate with scallions.

3. Meatloaf

4 servings (1 serving = ¼ meatloaf)

Ingredients
- 1 beaten egg
- 1 lb. 85% ground turkey or lean ground beef
- 2 tbsp. mayonnaise
- ½ cup breadcrumbs (panko)

Seasonings:
- 1 tsp. onion powder
- ½ tsp. red pepper flakes
- 1 tsp. garlic powder
- 1 tbsp. Worcestershire sauce, low-sodium
- 1 tsp. low sodium Better Than Bouillon Beef Base

Nutrition Per Serving

Calories	367 cal

Protein	25 g
Sodium	332 mg
Phosphorus	273 mg
Dietary Fiber	0.7 g
Potassium	460 mg

Directions
- Preheat the oven to 375 degrees F.
- In a medium-size bowl, combine all the ingredients (apart from turkey or ground beef) until well blended. Mix and add turkey and ground beef.
- Place the mixture in a meatloaf pan or shape it into an 8' x 4' elongated loaf or the meatloaf shape or form it into 2 individual meatloaves and place it on a tiny baking sheet tray.
- Cover it with aluminum foil and bake it for 20 minutes, after which remove the foil and cook for an extra 5 minutes. Turn off the oven and leave to rest in the oven before removing and delivering for 10 minutes.

4. Grilled Pork Chops and Peach Glaze

8 servings (1 serving = 4-oz. portion)

Ingredients
- 1 cup peach preserves
- 8 4-oz. pork chops, center-cut (choose boneless pork chops
- zest of 1 lime and ¼ cup lime juice
- 2 tbsp. cilantro
- 1 tsp. smoked paprika
- 1 tbsp. soy sauce, low-sodium
- ½ tsp. red pepper flakes
- 2 tsp. onion flakes, dried
- ¼ cup olive oil
- ½ tsp. black pepper

Nutrition Per Serving

Calories	357 cal
Protein	23 g
Sodium	158 mg
Phosphorus	188 mg
Dietary Fiber	0 g
Potassium	363 mg

Directions
- Heat the grill or switch to a high setting on the electric griddle.

- In a medium bowl, mix all the ingredients (apart from pork chops) until well blended.
- Remove a quarter of the mixture, set it aside, place the remaining marinade in a bag with pork chops and marinate it for 4 hours (overnight is better.
- Grill the pork chops from each side for 6-8 minutes.
- Glaze a last time before detaching from the grill and allow 7-10 minutes before serving to rest on a platter or plates.

5. Gnocchi and Chicken Dumplings

10 servings (1 serving = 1 cup portion)

Ingredients
- 1 lb. gnocchi
- 2 lb. chicken breast
- 1 tbsp. low sodium Better Than Bouillon Chicken Base
- ¼ cup light olive oil or grapeseed
- ½ cup finely diced, fresh celery
- 6 cups chicken stock, reduced-sodium
- ½ cup finely diced, fresh carrots
- 1 tsp. Italian seasoning
- ½ cup finely diced, fresh onions
- 1 teaspoon black pepper
- ¼ cup fresh, chopped parsley

Nutrition Per Serving

Calories	362 cal
Protein	28 g
Sodium	121 mg
Phosphorus	295 mg
Dietary Fiber	2 g
Potassium	485 mg

Directions
- Put the stockpot on the burner, add the oil, and set it to heat.
- Put the chicken in hot oil and cook until it is golden brown.
- Add the carrots, onions, and celery and cook until translucent, with the chicken. Add the chicken stock and let it cook for 20-30 minutes on high heat.
- Add the chicken bouillon, Italian seasoning, and black pepper, reduce the heat, mix. Add the gnocchi and cook, while stirring continuously, for 15 minutes.
- Remove it out from the burner, add parsley and eat.

6. Bourbon Glazed Skirt Steak

8 servings (1 serving = 3 oz.)

Ingredients
Bourbon Glaze:
- 3 tbsp. cubed and chilled, unsalted butter
- ¼ cup shallots, diced
- ¼ cup dark brown sugar
- 1 cup bourbon
- 1 tbsp. black pepper
- 2 tbsp. Dijon mustard

Skirt Steak:
- ½ tsp. dried oregano
- 2 tbsp. grapeseed oil
- 1 tsp. black pepper
- ½ tsp. smoked paprika
- 1 lb. skirt steak
- 1 tbsp. red wine vinegar

Nutrition Per Serving

Calories	409 cal
Protein	24 g
Sodium	152 mg
Phosphorus	171 mg
Dietary Fiber	0.5 g
Potassium	283 mg

Directions
Bourbon Glaze:
- On medium-high heat, brown the shallots in 1 tbsp. of butter in a small saucepan.
- Reduce the heat to a minimum, remove the pan from the burner, add the bourbon, and put back the saucepan to the burner.
- Cook for at least 10-15 minutes, or until around one third is reduced.
- Add mustard, black pepper, and brown sugar and whisk until bubbly.
- Switch off the heat and mix in the remaining 2 tsp. of cubed, cold butter, stir until well mixed.

Skirt Steak:
- In a sealable gallon-sized storage bag, combine the ingredients, add steaks, and mix well.
- Allow the steaks to be marinated in the bag for 30-45 minutes at room temperature.

- Remove the steaks from the bag, then grill each side for 15-20 minutes, and remove and put aside for 10 minutes to rest.
- Strip and serve with a sauce; otherwise, leave and brush with glaze and place in a preheated broiler for at least 4-6 minutes or until needed.

7. Chicken Pot Pie Stew

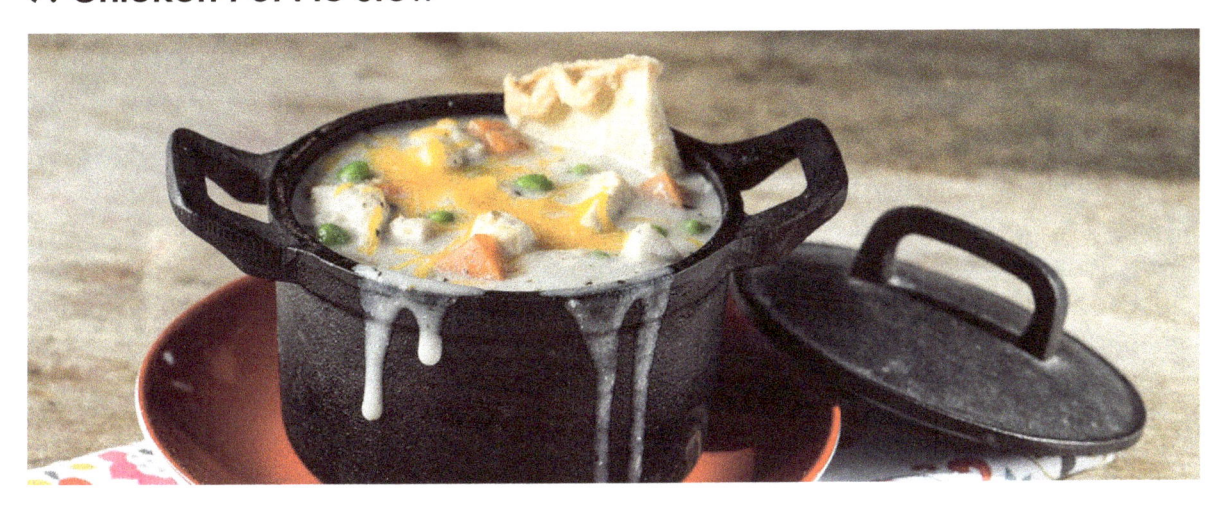

8 servings (1 serving = 1 cup portion)

Ingredients
- 2 cups chicken stock, low-sodium
- 1½ lb. boneless, skinless, natural fresh chicken breast
- ½ cup flour
- ½ cup fresh, diced onions
- ¼ cup canola oil
- ½ cup fresh, diced carrots
- ½ tsp. black pepper
- ¼ cup fresh, diced celery
- 2 tsp. low sodium, Better Than Bouillon Chicken Base
- 1 tbsp. Italian seasoning, sodium-free (e.g., McCormick)
- ½ cup heavy cream
- ½ cup thawed, fresh frozen sweet peas
- 1 cup Cheddar cheese, low-fat
- 1 frozen, cooked piecrust, broken into tiny pieces

Nutrition Per Serving

Calories	388 cal
Protein	26 g
Sodium	424 mg
Phosphorus	290 mg
Dietary Fiber	2 g

| Potassium | 209 mg |

Directions
- Pound chicken to tenderize and slice into tiny cubes.
- Put the chicken and stock in a wide stockpot and cook for 30 minutes on medium-high heat. Meanwhile, till well blended, mix the flour and oil.
- Then pour and stir slowly into the mixture of chicken broth till slightly thickened. For 15 minutes, reduce the heat to medium-low.
- Add the onions, carrots, black pepper, celery, bouillon, and Italian seasoning. For an extra 15 minutes, cook.
- Turn the heat off and add the cream and peas. Mix until well blended. Serve in the mugs and top as a garnish equal quantity of cheese and piecrust.

8. BBQ Baby Back Ribs, Sauce-less

12 servings (1 serving = 1/3 pound or 1/6 slab bone-in raw weight)

Ingredients
- 1 portion of rub
- 12 frozen or fresh, mini-ears corn on the cob
- 2 slabs baby back ribs (about 3½ pounds)

BBQ Spice Rub (mix all the ingredients):
- 1 tsp. black pepper
- 1 cup dark brown sugar, packed
- 1 tsp. smoked paprika
- 2 tsp. dark chili powder
- 1 tsp. red pepper flakes
- 2 tsp. onion flakes, dehydrated
- 2 tsp. granulated garlic

Nutrition Per Serving

Calories	324 cal
Protein	18 g
Sodium	102 mg
Phosphorus	198 mg
Dietary Fiber	2.3 g
Potassium	453 mg

Directions
- Preheat the oven to 400° F.
- Rub down both the slabs of ribs with rub mixture on both sides.

- Place the ribs in a rack-lined wire tray. Cover with aluminum foil firmly and bake for 1 1/2 to 2 hours.
- Take off the foil and remove it from the oven. Set the ribs aside using tongs. Drain the liquid from the pan and bring the ribs back on the tray.
- Cook for 15 minutes or until the perfect crispness if desired.
- Leave for 5 to 10 minutes to rest, then cut and eat.
- Prefer a microwave-safe 9" x 9" casserole tray to microwave the corn on the cob. Stand in the dish the mini-ears of corn at the end. Onto the dish, add around 1/2 inch of water. With the plastic wrap, cover firmly. Microwave for 5-7 minutes on high.

9. Roast Pork Loin With Tart and Sweet Apple Stuffing

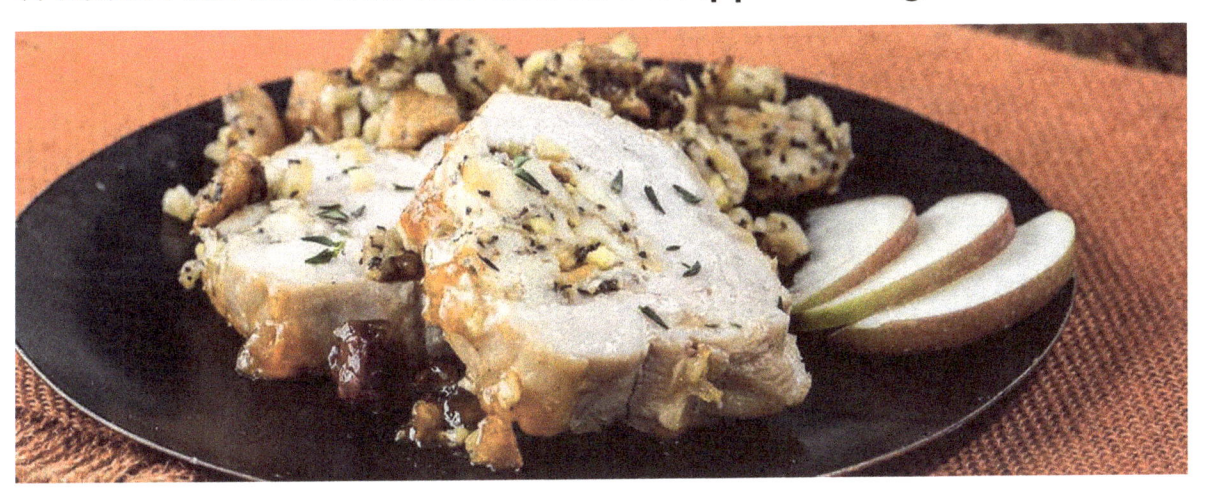

6 servings (1 serving = 2.5–3 oz. or 1/6 loin)

Ingredients
Cherry Marmalade Glaze:
- 1/4 cup apple juice
- 1/8 tsp. nutmeg
- 1/2 cup orange marmalade, sugar-free
- 1/8 tsp. cinnamon
- 1/4 cup cherries, dried

Apple Stuffing:
- 2 cups Hawaiian rolls, cubed and packed
- 2 tbsp. canola oil
- 2 tbsp. unsalted butter
- 1/2 cup finely diced Macintosh, Honey Crisp apple, or Granny Smith
- 2 tbsp. celery, finely diced
- 1/2 cup chicken stock, low-sodium
- 2 tbsp. onions, finely diced

- 1 tsp. black pepper
- ½ teaspoon dried thyme or 1 tbsp. fresh thyme

Roast Pork Loin:
- 2 butcher twine of 18-inch pieces
- 1 lb. Hormel natural pork loin, boneless

Nutrition Per Serving

Calories	263 cal
Protein	14 g
Sodium	137 mg
Phosphorus	154 mg
Dietary Fiber	1 g
Potassium	275 mg

Directions

Cherry Marmalade Glaze:
- On a medium-high flame, blend all the glaze ingredients in a medium saucepan till the marmalade is melted and begins to simmer. Turn the heat off and put it aside.
- Preheat the oven to 400° F.
- Sauté all the ingredients in canola oil in a broad sauté pan over medium-high heat for 2-3 minutes, except chicken stock.
- Add the chicken stock slowly till it is moist and not too wet. (Based on how much juice is extracted from the apples while cooking, you do not need it all.)
- Remove from the heat to room temperature and relax.
- Meanwhile, down the length of the loin, slice five slits about 1 inch apart, forming many pockets.
- With about 2 tsp. of stuffing, fill each pocket with (there should be a little leftover).
- To hold the stuffing in place, tie one long piece of twine across the length of the loin, then tie additional twine around the shorter length as required.
- On a baking sheet plate, put the remaining stuffing, place the tied stuffed pork on the top and bake at 400 ° F for 45 minutes or till you hit an internal temperature of 160 ° F.
- Spoon on the glaze of dried cherry marmalade, switch off the oven heat and let it cool for 10-15 minutes in the oven. Cut the pork loin, then slice into pieces and eat.

10. Asparagus and Spaghetti Carbonara

6 servings (1 serving = 1 cup)

Ingredients

- 1 cup diced, fresh onions
- 2 tsp. canola oil
- 1 cup heavy cream
- 1 large, beaten egg
- 3 cups spiral noodle pasta (cooked), about 1 ½ cups raw, cooked al dente
- ¼ cup chicken stock, low-sodium
- 3 tbsp. Parmesan cheese, shredded
- 1 tsp. black pepper, freshly cracked coarse
- 2 cups chopped, fresh asparagus, about 1" long pieces
- 3 tbsp. meatless bacon bits
- ½ cup chopped, fresh scallions

Nutrition Per Serving

Calories	304 cal
Protein	9 g
Sodium	141 mg
Phosphorus	143 mg
Dietary Fiber	5.4 mg
Potassium	287 mg

Directions
- Heat oil and sauté the onions in a large nonstick pan over medium-high heat till lightly browned.
- In the meantime, whisk the cream and the eggs in a small bowl till entirely mixed.
- Reduce the heat to medium and add the mixture of cream into the onions, stirring frequently for about 4 to 6 minutes with a wooden spoon till it begins to thicken.
- Add the pasta, stock, black pepper, and asparagus and mix for another 3-4 minutes or till thoroughly warmed.
- Turn off the flame and spill the carbonara it into a serving dish. Top and serve with bacon bits, cheese, and scallions.

11. Cabbage, Onion Sweet Pepper Medley

4 servings (1 Serving = ¼ Recipe)

Ingredients
- ½ cup green bell pepper, fresh
- ½ cup red bell pepper, fresh
- ½ cup fresh, chopped onions
- ½ cup yellow bell pepper, fresh
- 3 tbsp. white vinegar
- 2 cups fresh, shredded cabbage

- 1 ½ tsp. brown sugar
- 1 tbsp. canola oil
- 1 ½ tsp. pepper
- 1 ½ tsp. Dijon mustard

Nutrition Per Serving

Calories	70 cal
Protein	1 g
Sodium	52 mg
Phosphorus	29 mg
Dietary Fiber	2 g
Potassium	208 mg

Directions
- Cut the bell peppers into thin slices that are 2 inches long.
- Combine the onion, bell peppers, and cabbage in a broad nonstick skillet and toss gently.
- In a jar, mix the vinegar and other ingredients, firmly cover, and vigorously shake.
- Add to the mixture of vegetables, stirring softly.
- Sauté till the cabbage is tender, on medium heat and mix periodically.

12. Adobo Marinated Tilapia Tapas

12 servings (1 serving = 4 wonton cups)

Ingredients
- Nonstick cooking spray
- 48 wonton wrappers, small
- 6 pieces of tilapia filets (3-oz.)

Adobo Sauce:
- 1 tbsp. oregano
- 3 tbsp. Spanish paprika
- ¼ cup olive oil, extra-virgin
- 1 tsp. black pepper
- 3 tbsp. chopped, fresh cilantro
- ½ cup red wine vinegar
- 1 tsp. red pepper flakes

Slaw Mix:
- 1 tbsp. chopped, fresh garlic
- ½ cup mayonnaise
- 4 cups fresh, shredded slaw mix cabbage

- ¼ cup lemon juice
- ¼ cup fresh, rough cut, cilantro leaves
- ¼ cup fresh, sliced thin on the bias, green scallions

Nutrition Per Serving

Calories	254 cal
Protein	13 g
Sodium	272 mg
Phosphorus	116 mg
Dietary Fiber	2 g
Potassium	268 mg

Directions
- Preheat the oven to 400° F.
- Mix all the adobo ingredients until well blended and put aside.
- Marinate the fish fillets for 30 minutes in half a cup of adobe sauce.
- Slightly oil the baking sheet tray and bake the fish at 400° F for 15 minutes, turning halfway. Take it out of the oven and put it aside.
- In a medium-sized bowl, add the mayo, garlic, the remaining adobo sauce, cilantro, and scallions until well combined. Add the cabbage and blend gently till it is coated.
- Use cooking spray to spray a mini muffin pan. Us one wonton wrapper to line the muffin cups.
- Bake at 350 degrees F for 5 minutes, let it cool and pick the crispy wontons from the pan.
- Place equal servings of fish on wontons (break or cut into 48 pieces) and cover with equal quantities of slaw mix. Garnish with leaves of cilantro and eat.

13. Crunchy and Sweet and Coleslaw

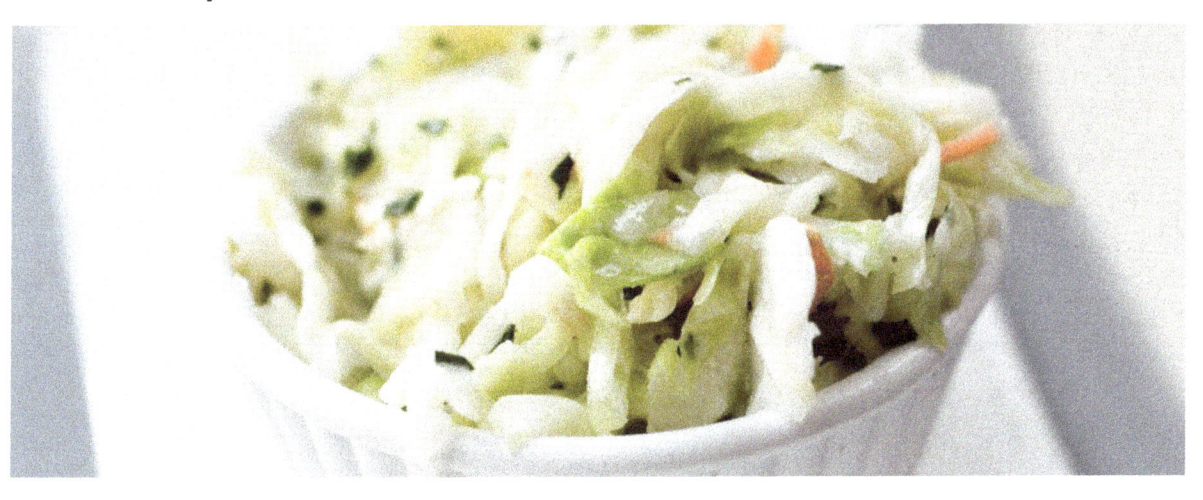

12 servings (1 serving = ½ cup)

Ingredients
- ½ cup chopped, sweet onion
- 6 cups cabbage, shredded
- 1 tsp. yellow prepared mustard
- 1 cup canola oil
- 1 cup of sugar
- ½ cup of rice vinegar
- 1 tsp. celery seed

Nutrition Per Serving

Calories	244 cal
Protein	1 g
Sodium	12 mg
Phosphorus	13 mg
Dietary Fiber	1 g
Potassium	73 mg

Directions
- Mix the shredded cabbage in a large bowl with the chopped onion.
- Mix all other ingredients in a blender till well blended.
- Pour the dressing over onion and cabbage. Mix and refrigerate.
- Serve it cold.

14. Red Cabbage Casserole

8 servings (1 serving = ½ cup)

Ingredients
- 1 cup chopped, fresh onion
- 1 tbsp. butter, unsalted
- 1 shredded, fresh medium red cabbage (about 4 cups)
- ¼ cup red wine vinegar
- ¼ tsp. black pepper, ground
- 3 cups fresh cored, peeled, sliced apples
- 2 tbsp. brown sugar
- ¼ cup of water

Nutrition Per Serving

Calories	79 cal
Protein	1 g
Sodium	13 mg
Phosphorus	23 mg

| Dietary Fiber | 2 g |
| Potassium | 161 mg |

Directions
- Preheat the oven to 300° F.
- Grease a broad dish of casserole.
- In a big bowl, combine all the ingredients, excluding butter. Put them in the casserole bowl. Dot with the butter.
- Cover the casserole dish and simmer for 2 1/2 hours at 300 ° F.

15. Mediterranean Green Beans

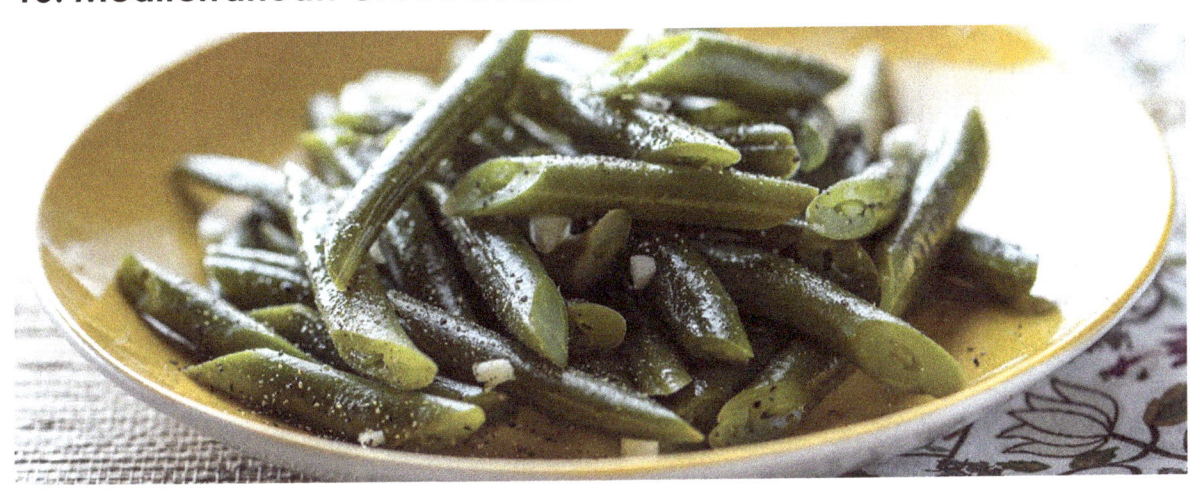

4 servings (1 serving = 1 cup)

Ingredients
- ¾ cup water
- 1 lb. green beans, cut to 1 to 2-inch pieces
- 3 fresh, minced garlic cloves
- 2 ½ tsp. olive oil
- 1/8 tsp. black pepper
- 3 tbsp. lemon juice, fresh

Nutrition Per Serving

Calories	71 cal
Protein	2 g
Sodium	2 mg
Phosphorus	37 mg
Dietary Fiber	3.7 g
Potassium	186 mg

Directions

- In a big, nonstick skillet, bring the water to a boil; add beans, cook for 3 minutes, and then drain and set aside.
- Over a medium-high flame, heat the skillet and add oil; add the beans and garlic, and sauté for at least 1 minute.
- Mix in the pepper and juice and sauté for 1 minute.
- TIP: Instead of salt, use lemon juice to bring out the food's flavor.

16. Zucchini Sauté

6 servings (1 serving = ½ cup)

Ingredients
- 1 cup whole milk
- 3-4 sliced, medium-size zucchini (about 4 cups)
- ¼ cup Parmesan cheese, grated
- ½ cup flour
- ½ tsp. fresh thyme
- Pepper to taste
- ½ tsp. fresh basil
- 2 tbsp. vegetable oil
- ½ tsp. tarragon, fresh

Nutrition Per Serving

Calories	121 cal
Protein	4 g
Sodium	75 mg
Phosphorus	91 mg
Dietary Fiber	1.5 g
Potassium	374 mg

Directions
- Place the zucchini in the milk to soak.
- In a bowl, mix the parmesan cheese, pepper, and flour, then add herbs.
- In a big skillet, heat the vegetable oil.
- Dip the zucchini into a mixture of herbs and cheese.
- Sauté. Then serve it hot.

17. Smothered Pork Chops with Sautéed Greens

6 servings (1 serving = 1 pork chop, 1/6 sautéed greens)

Ingredients
Smothered Pork Chops:
- 1 tbsp. black pepper
- 6 center-cut, natural, bone-in pork loin chops
- 2 tsp. onion powder, granulated
- 2 tsp. paprika
- 1 cup and 2 tbsp. flour
- 2 tsp. garlic powder, granulated
- 2 cups beef stock, low-sodium
- ½ cup canola oil
- ½ cup fresh, sliced on the bias, scallions
- 1 ½ cups sliced, fresh onions

Sautéed Greens:
- 2 tbsp. olive oil
- 8 cups fresh chopped and blanched collard greens
- ¼ cup finely diced onions
- 1 tbsp. butter, unsalted
- 1 tsp. red pepper flakes, crushed
- 1 tbsp. chopped, fresh garlic
- 1 tsp. vinegar (optional)
- 1 tsp. black pepper

Nutrition Per Serving

Calories	464 cal
Protein	27 g
Sodium	108 mg
Phosphorus	289 mg
Dietary Fiber	1.3 g
Potassium	604 mg

Directions
Preheat the oven to 350° F.

Pork Chops:
- Mix in the paprika, black pepper, garlic powder, and onion powder. Season both the sides of the pork chops with half of the mixture and combine the other half with 1 cup of flour.
- For later, save 2 tbsp. of the flour mix.
- Coat the pork chops lightly with the seasoned flour.

- Heat the oil in a big Dutch oven on medium-high or use an oven-ready sauté pan (with no rubber handles).
- Fry the pork chops on each side for 2-4 minutes or till crispness is needed. Take it out of the pan and pour off all but 2 tbsp of oil.
- Cook the onions for around 4-6 minutes, until translucent. Stir in 2 tbsp. of the reserved flour and blend well for around 1 minute with the onions.
- Add the beef stock slowly and mix until it thickens.
- Place the pork chops back in the pan and coat them with sauce. Wrap or cover with a foil and cook in the oven at 350° F for at least 30-45 minutes.
- Remove from the oven and set to rest before serving for at least 5-10 minutes.

Sautéed Greens:
- Add the greens to boiling water for at least 30 seconds to blanch the greens.
- Strain the boiling water and transfer it quickly to a bowl of water and ice.
- Let the greens cool, strain and dry, after which set aside.
- Melt the oil and butter together in a large sauté pan over medium-high flame. Add the garlic and onions and cook for about 4-6 minutes, till slightly browned.
- Add the collard greens and the red and black pepper, cook on high heat for 5-8 minutes, stirring continuously.
- Remove from flame; add vinegar, if required, and stir.

18. Crunchy Lemon Herbed Chicken

4 servings (1 serving = 3-oz. portion)

Ingredients
- 4 tbsp. chilled, unsalted butter
- 6 2-oz. chicken tenders
- zest of 1 lemon or ¼ cup of lemon juice
- ½ cup breadcrumbs (panko)
- 1 tbsp. chopped, fresh oregano
- 3 tbsp. water (2 tbsp. for finishing the sauce and 1 tbsp. for the egg wash)
- 1 egg yolk
- 1 tbsp. chopped fresh thyme
- 1 tbsp. chopped fresh basil

Nutrition Per Serving

Calories	277 cal
Protein	22 g
Sodium	141 mg
Phosphorus	226 mg

| Dietary Fiber | 0.9 g |
| Potassium | 347 mg |

Directions

- On a medium-low flame, preheat 2 tbsp of butter.
- Add 1 lemon zest and half the herbs to the breadcrumbs, then save the remainder for the lemon sauce.
- Beat the yolk of an egg with 1 tbsp. of water.
- Place the chicken tenders between 2 plastic wraps and beat till thin and not ripped, with the mallet's small groove side.
- Dip the chicken till coated in the mixture of egg wash and then a mixture of herbed breadcrumbs. Set aside them.
- On medium heat, preheat 2 tbsp of butter.
- Place the breaded chicken in the sauté pan.
- Cook the chicken from each side for about 2-3 minutes.
- Take the chicken out and place it on the baking sheet pan to settle. Add the lemon juice and the remaining herbs to the same pan and heat again till simmering.
- Turn off the heat; add to the sauce the remaining 2 tbsp. of butter, stir vigorously.
- Slice the chicken.
- Place the sliced chicken, sprinkle the sauce on the top, and add the garnishes on a plate.

19. Orzo Salad

8 servings (1 serving = ½ cup)

Ingredients

- 1 cup cranberries, dried
- 4 cups chilled, cooked orzo (dried orzo about 1 2/3 cups)
- ¼ cup olive oil, extra-virgin
- 2 cups fresh, diced apple
- ¼ cup chopped, blanched almonds
- ½ tsp. black pepper, freshly ground
- ¼ cup lemon juice, fresh
- ½ cup blue cheese, crumbled
- 2 tbsp. chopped, fresh basil

Nutrition Per Serving

Calories	289 cal
Protein	6 g
Sodium	100 mg
Phosphorus	94 mg

| Dietary Fiber | 3 g |
| Potassium | 127 mg |

Directions
- Add the ingredients, excluding almonds and blue cheese, into a medium-sized bowl, mix gently until well combined.
- Move the mixture to a serving plate, cover it with the almonds, and crumble blue cheese and serve.

20. Chili Cornbread Casserole

8 servings (1 serving = 8 oz.)

Ingredients
Chili:
- ½ cup diced onions
- 1 lb. ground beef
- 2 tbsp. chopped jalapeño peppers
- ¼ cup diced celery
- 1 tbsp. chili powder
- ½ cup chopped green or red peppers
- 2 tbsp. onion flakes, dried
- 1 tbsp. cumin
- 1 tbsp. garlic powder, granulated
- ½ cup tomato sauce (no salt added)
- 1 tsp. black pepper
- ¼ cup reduced-sodium French's Worcestershire sauce
- ¼ cup of water
- 1 cup shredded cheddar cheese
- 1 cup dried and rinsed kidney beans

Cornbread:
- ¾ cup flour
- ¼ cup cornmeal
- ¾ cup milk
- ½ tsp. cream of tartar
- ¼ tsp. baking soda
- 1 beaten egg
- ½ cup of sugar
- ¼ cup canola oil
- 1½ tbsp. melted, unsalted butter

Nutrition Per Serving

Calories	392 cal
Protein	17 g
Sodium	335 mg
Phosphorus	239 mg
Dietary Fiber	2.9 g
Potassium	441 mg

Directions
- Brown the ground beef in a broad saucepan with jalapeños, bell peppers, celery, and onions. Drain the oil in excess. Add the garlic powder, chili powder, onion flakes, tomato sauce, cumin, black pepper, Worcestershire sauce, beans, and water. For an extra 10 minutes, cook. Remove from the flame and pour into a baking pan of 9" x 9" and then layer the cheese.
- Mix the flour, cornmeal, baking soda, tartar cream and sugar in a medium-size bowl.
- Beat the egg, oil, melted butter, and milk in a small bowl. Fold together the flour mixture and the egg mixture (you might see some lumps, that is okay, do not overbeat).
- Pour the mixture over the chili and bake uncovered for 25 minutes, then covered at 350 ° F for 20 minutes and then switch off the oven and allow to rest for 5 minutes.

21. Lemon Chicken, Slow-Cooked

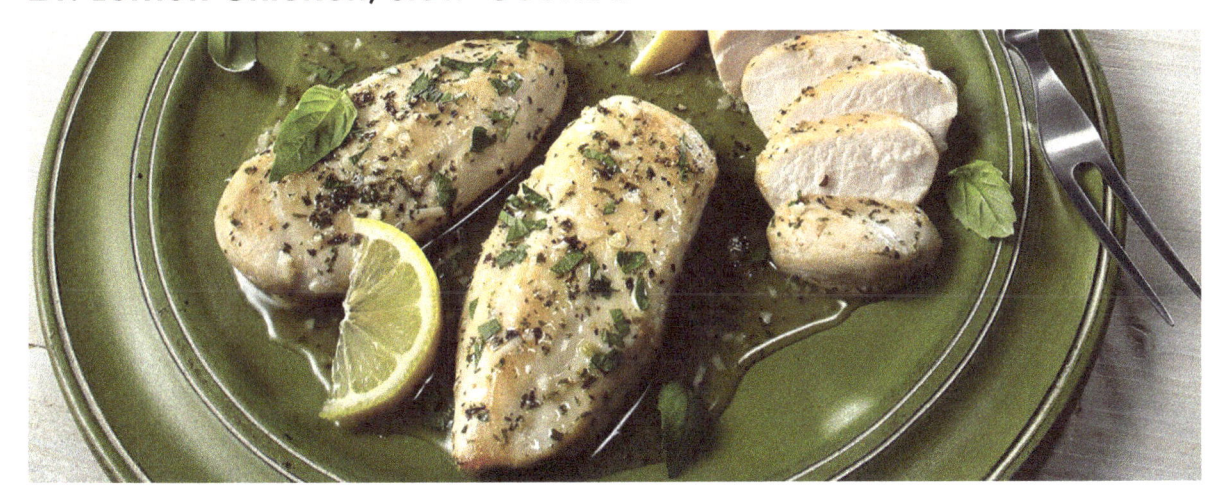

4 servings (1 serving = 4 oz.)

Ingredients
- ¼ tsp. ground black pepper
- 1 tsp. oregano, dried
- 1 lb. skinless, boneless chicken breast
- 2 tbsp. unsalted butter
- 1 tsp. chopped fresh basil

- ¼ cup water
- ¼ cup low sodium chicken broth
- 2 minced cloves garlic
- 1 tbsp. lemon juice

Nutrition Per Serving

Calories	197 cal
Protein	26 g
Sodium	57 mg
Phosphorus	251 mg
Dietary Fiber	0.3 g
Potassium	412 mg

Directions

- In a small bowl, combine the ground black pepper and oregano. Rub the mixture on chicken.
- In a medium-size skillet on medium flame, melt the butter. In the melting butter, brown the chicken and then switch the chicken to a slow cooker.
- In the skillet, place the water, chicken broth, garlic, and lemon juice and garlic. Get it to a boil, so the browned pieces are loosened from the skillet. Place over the chicken.
- Cover the slow cooker for 21/2 hours on maximum or 5 hours on low.
- Combine the basil and baste the chicken. Cover and cook for a further 15-30 minutes or till the chicken is tender.

22. Green Bean Casserole

6 servings (1 serving = 3 oz.)

Ingredients

- 2 tbsp. hot sauce
- 12 oz of String green beans, Fresh
- ½ cup crushed, plain tortilla chips, unsalted
- 2 tbsp. unsalted, melted butter
- ¼ cup crumbled or shredded, sharp or gorgonzola cheddar cheese
- 2 tbsp. chopped green onions
- ½ cup breadcrumbs

Nutrition Per Serving

Calories	122 cal
Protein	4 g
Sodium	221 mg

Phosphorus	49 mg
Dietary Fiber	2.4 g
Potassium	219 mg

Directions

- Preheat the oven to 375 degrees F.
- Chop the green beans into 2" pieces (steam in a microwave-safe plate for 5-7 minutes, damp, soggy paper towel)
- Mix the hot sauce with the cut string green beans. Pour the mixture into the casserole dish.
- In a small bowl, combine the remaining ingredients. Scatter mixture uniformly over the string green beans, then bake uncovered, the green bean casserole in an oven for 12-15 minutes or till crispness is required, then serve.

23. Beef Stroganoff with Egg Noodles

6 servings (1 serving = 10 oz.)

Ingredients

- 1 beaten egg
- 1 cup finely diced onions
- ¼ cup breadcrumbs
- 2 tbsp. reduced-sodium, French's Worcestershire sauce
- 1 tbsp. tomato sauce (no salt added)
- 1 tbsp. mayonnaise
- 3 tbsp. canola oil
- 1 lb. ground beef
- 3 cups of water
- 2 tbsp. flour
- 4 tsp. reduced-sodium, Better Than Bouillon beef
- 1 tsp. ground black pepper
- 2 tbsp. chives
- ¼ cup sour cream
- 2 tbsp. unsalted, cubed, and cold butter
- ½ package of wide, cooked egg noodles, (12oz package)
- 1 tbsp. chopped rosemary
- ¼ cup parsley

Nutrition Per Serving

| Calories | 490 cal |

Protein	20 g
Sodium	598 mg
Phosphorus	230 mg
Dietary Fiber	1.8 mg
Potassium	423 mg

Directions

- Mix half of the black pepper and the ingredients (first six) in a wide bowl. Add beef and mix properly. Make 16 meatballs of the same size.
- Cook the stroganoff meatballs in a large saucepan over medium heat until browned. Pull all the meatballs to one side by adding the flour and oil to the pan, stir well until mixed properly. Add the remaining black pepper, bouillon and water and mix for about 10 minutes until thickened.
- Turn off the heat and add the chives and sour cream, then serve over the egg noodles.

Pasta:

- Add the egg noodles with 2 tbsp. of water to the large sauté pan/pot, heat and stir till warm, and then turn off the heat. Stir in the parsley, rosemary, and butter till everything is balanced.

24. Slow-Cooked Pulled Pork, Hawaiian-Style

16 servings (1 serving = 4 oz.)

Ingredients

- ½ tsp. ground black pepper
- 4 lb. pork roast
- 1 tsp. onion powder
- ½ tsp. paprika
- 2 tbsp. liquid smoke
- ½ tsp. garlic powder

Nutrition Per Serving

Calories	285 mg
Protein	20 g
Sodium	54 mg
Phosphorus	230 mg
Dietary Fiber	0 g
Potassium	380 mg

Directions

- In a small bowl, mix the paprika, black pepper, garlic powder, and onion together.

- Rub both sides of the pork with the seasoning mixture. Put the pork in a crock-pot or a slow cooker. Sprinkle with the liquid smoke.
- To weigh 1/4-1/2" deep, add sufficient water to the crock-pot or slow cooker. Cook for 4-5 hours on high.
- Using two forks, shred the meat and separate pork from the cooking liquid.
- **Optional:** Garnish with radishes or sliced pickled red onions.
- **Tip:** Marinate four sliced radishes or one sliced red onion in 1/3 cup of white vinegar and 1/4 tsp. of sugar for an hour for radishes or quick pickled red onions. Rinse and use as a garnish.
- **Note:** There are several ways to use shredded or pulled pork. Add it to a soup, serve it over rice, or make a high-protein breakfast by placing it in scrambled eggs.

25. Herb Crusted Roast Leg of Lamb

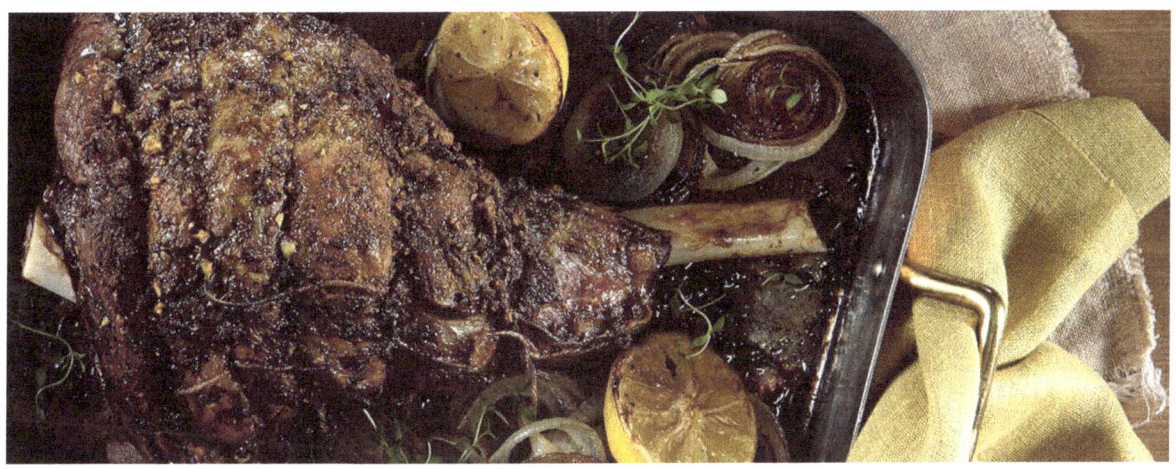

12 servings (1 serving = 4 oz.)

Ingredients
- 3 tbsp. lemon juice
- 1 4-lb. leg of lamb
- 2 minced cloves garlic
- ½ cup vermouth, dry
- 1 tbsp. curry powder
- 1 cup sliced onions
- ½ tsp. ground black pepper

Nutrition Per Serving

Calories	292 mg
Protein	24 g
Sodium	157 mg
Phosphorus	232 mg
Dietary Fiber	0 g

| Potassium | 419 mg |

Directions

- Preheat the oven to 400° F.
- Place the lamb's leg in the roasting pan. Sprinkle with 1 tsp. lemon juice.
- Use 2 tsp. of lemon juice and the remaining spices to make the paste. Rub the mixture or paste onto the lamb.
- Roast the lamb for 30 minutes in the oven at 400° F.
- Drain the fat and add the onions and vermouth.
- Reduce the heat to 325 ° F and simmer for an extra 1¾-2 hours. Baste the lamb's leg frequently. Remove from the oven when the internal temperature is 145 ° F and leave to rest for 3 minutes at least before serving.

26. Herb-Crusted Pork Loin

14 servings (1 serving = 4 oz.)

Ingredients

- 2 tbsp. low sodium, soy sauce
- 1 pork loin roast, boneless (3½ pounds)
- 2 tbsp. fennel seed
- 2 tbsp. anise seed
- 2 tbsp. dill seed
- 2 tbsp. caraway seed

Nutrition Per Serving

Calories	224 cal
Protein	24 g
Sodium	134 mg
Phosphorus	225 mg
Dietary Fiber	1.0 g
Potassium	405 mg

Directions

- Apply soy sauce over the roast until all over is coated. Stir together the fennel, anise seed, dill seed, and caraway in a 13' x 10' x 1' baking pan. To coat equally, roll pork roast in seeds. Wrap the meat in a foil; put it in the fridge for 2 hours or overnight.
- Preheat the oven to 325°F and remove the foil. In a shallow open roasting pan, put the meat fat side up on the rack. Insert the meat thermometer such that the tip is in the middle of the thickest section.
- In the baking pan, roast pork loin for 35-40 minutes per lb. When roast is done, the meat thermometer should record 145 ° F. Let it rest for 3 minutes. Slice and serve.

27. Black Bean Burger and Cilantro Slaw

6 servings (1 serving = 1 burger)

Ingredients
- ½ cup bulgur wheat (to prepare mix ½ cup bulgur wheat with ½ cup hot water and set aside for at least 30 minutes)
- ½ cup low sodium, drained, rinsed, mashed, and dried black beans
- 1 tsp. granulated garlic
- 1 tsp. ground black pepper
- 1 tbsp. Reduced sodium, French's Worcestershire sauce
- ½ tsp. smoked paprika
- 1 tbsp. reduced-sodium, Better Than Bouillon beef
- 1 tsp. onion flakes
- ¼ cup scallions
- ½ cup onions (sautéed until translucent)
- 3 cups slaw mix, 10-oz. bag
- 2 tbsp. flour
- 2 tbsp. cilantro
- ¼ cup balsamic vinegar
- 2 tbsp. canola oil for searing
- 2 tbsp. sesame oil
- zest of one lime
- ¼ cup lime juice
- 6 hamburger rolls
- ¼ cup mayonnaise

Nutrition Per Serving

Calories	380 cal
Protein	9 g
Sodium	520 mg
Phosphorus	129 mg
Dietary Fiber	5 g
Potassium	313 mg

Directions
- Preheat the oven to 400° F.
- Combine bulgur wheat, black beans, ground black pepper, smoked paprika, granulated garlic, onion flakes, Worcestershire sauce, beef bouillon, half a cup of scallions and onions in a medium-sized bowl.
- Mold about half a cup of the mixture into the burgers and refrigerate or freeze until firmly formed (not frozen).

- Make a vinaigrette by combining sesame oil, 1 tbsp. of cilantro, lime juice and vinegar together. Add all but 2 tbsp. of vinaigrette to the slaw mix in a small bowl and whisk gently, then put aside in the fridge.
- Add the mayonnaise and the remaining 2 tbsp. of vinaigrette to another small bowl and set aside.
- Dust the flour on the black bean burgers and remove the excess. Put on the pre-sprayed pan and also spray the burger tops. Bake for at least 14 minutes and flip around burgers halfway through.
- Toast rolls and adds an equal quantity of mayo. Add the black bean burger and cover with around 1/4 cup (or the quantity you want) of slaw.
- **Optional:** Gently grill, on medium-high, the black bean burger with the canola oil on either side for about 3-4 minutes if you are in a rush.

28. Egg, Bacon, and Shrimp Grit Cakes with Cheese Sauce

6 servings (1 serving = 7 oz.)

Ingredients
- 2 tbsp. unsalted butter
- 4 beaten eggs
- 4 slices bacon, cubed in ½-inch pieces, reduced-sodium
- ½ cup diced onions
- 1 tsp. Old Bay Seasoning, low sodium
- 12 16/20 count, chopped, peeled, raw, and deveined shrimp
- ½ cup chicken stock (no added salt)
- ¼ cup chopped chives
- 1 cup milk (½ cup for sauce and ½ cup of grits)
- 2 tsp. reduced-sodium, Better Than Bouillon chicken flavor
- 2 tbsp. canola oil
- ½ cup grits
- ½ tsp. smoked paprika
- ½ tsp. ground black pepper
- ¼ cup Monterey jack, provolone, or Havarti cheese
- ¼ cup sharp, shredded cheddar cheese
- 1 tbsp. flour
- ¼ cup canola oil

Nutrition Per Serving

Calories	390 cal
Protein	15 g
Sodium	831 mg

Phosphorus	240 mg
Dietary Fiber	1.1 g
Potassium	230 mg

Directions

- In a broad nonstick sauté pan, heat the canola oil and scramble the eggs until slightly cooked, but not too dry in a medium-sized bowl, set aside. Add the butter to the pan and sauté the bacon, onions, shrimp, half of the chives, and Old Bay until the shrimp is lightly pink. Place them in the same bowl as the eggs.
- Add milk, chicken stock, grits and bouillon using the same pan and cook till done as per package instructions. Turn the heat off and fold the mixture of bacon, shrimp, and egg into grits in the pan. Pour the mixture into a 9" x 9" baking pan that is lightly oiled and spread until even; after that, cover and refrigerate till firm.
- Remove and slice into 6 squares. Heat the milk (for sauce) in a saucepan until warm, and whisk in the black pepper, cheese, paprika and the remaining chives until they are melted. Place aside the sauce.
- Heat ½ of the canola oil in a wide sauté pan. Dust the grit cakes gently with flour and sauté until they are golden brown. Plate over the top with similar quantities of smoky cheese sauce.

29. Cranberry Pork Roast

12 servings (1 serving = 4 oz.)

Ingredients

- ½ tsp. salt
- 4 lb. pork roast, center-cut
- 1 cup chopped cranberries
- ⅛ tsp. nutmeg
- 1 tsp. black pepper
- ¼ cup honey
- 1 tbsp. brown sugar
- ⅛ tsp. ground cloves
- 1 tsp. orange peel (zest), grated

Nutrition Per Serving

Calories	287 cal
Protein	30 g
Sodium	190 mg

Phosphorus	240 mg
Dietary Fiber	0.4 g
Potassium	406 mg

Directions
- Sprinkle the pork roast with pepper and salt. Put it in a crock-pot or slow cooker.
- Add the rest of the ingredients and pour over roast.
- Cover and simmer for 8-10 hours on low.
- From the crock-pot or slow cooker, cut the roast and slice it into 24 pieces. Cover it with a spoonful of drippings.

30. Bavarian Pot Roast

12 servings (1 serving = 4 oz.)

Ingredients
- 1 tsp. vegetable oil
- 3 lb. beef chuck roast
- ½ tsp. pepper
- ½ tsp. ground fresh ginger
- 2 cups sliced apples
- 3 whole cloves
- ½ cup water or apple juice
- ½ cup sliced onions
- 4 tbsp. water
- 4 tbsp. flour
- Optional garnish: apple slices, fresh

Nutrition Per Serving

Calories	313 cal
Protein	22 g
Sodium	73 mg
Phosphorus	202 mg
Dietary Fiber	1 g
Potassium	373 mg

Directions
- Trim the extra fat off the beef roast. Rinse and dry. Apply oil on the roast's top, and sprinkle with the pepper and ginger, then apply the entire cloves to the roast. After that, in a hot pan with oil, sear the pot roast on both sides.
- In a slow cooker or crock-pot, put the onions and apples. Add the pot roast and spill juice of apple over the whole roast.
- Cover and cook for 10-12 hours on low, or at least 5-6 hours on high.

- Take the roast off the slow cooker. Put it aside, keep it warm through.
- Strain the juices from the pot roast and drain them back into the slow cooker. To lessen the liquid and thicken it, turn the heat to high.
- Using flour and water, create a smooth paste; after that, add it to the slow cooker, mixing while you combine.
- Cover and simmer until it thickens. Just before serving, spill over the roast.
- Optional: Garnish with slices of fresh apples.

31. Spicy Beef Stir-Fry

4 servings (1 serving = 1 cup)

Ingredients
- ¼ tsp. sesame oil
- 2 tbsp. separated corn-starch
- 2 tbsp. water, separated
- ½ tsp. sugar
- 3 tbsp. canola oil, separated
- 1 large beaten egg
- 1 sliced, green bell pepper
- 12 oz. Sliced beef round tip
- ¼ tsp. red chili pepper, ground
- 1 cup sliced onions
- 2 tsp. reduced-sodium, soy sauce
- 1 tbsp. sherry
- Optional garnish: parsley

Nutrition Per Serving

Calories	261 cal
Protein	21 g
Sodium	169 mg
Phosphorus	167 mg
Dietary Fiber	1.5 g
Potassium	313 mg

Directions
- Whisk 1 tbsp. of corn-starch, 1 tbsp. of water, 1 big egg, and 1 tbsp. of canola oil in a large bowl and add the beef. For 20 minutes, marinate.
- Combine the remaining corn-starch and water in a separate bowl. After that, put it aside.
- In a skillet, heat the rest of the 2 tbsp. of canola oil and add the mixture of meat to it. Cook till the browning of the meat begins.

- Add the green bell peppers, chili pepper and onion. Add the sherry and stir fry for a minute. Add soy sauce, sesame oil and sugar.
- Thicken with a mixture of corn-starch and water.
- **Optional:** Garnish the beef stir-fry with the parsley.

32. Zesty Orange Tilapia

4 servings (1 serving = 4 oz.)

Ingredients
- 1 cup julienned carrots
- 16 oz. tilapia
- 1 tsp. ground black pepper
- ½ cup sliced, green onions
- ¾ cup julienned celery
- 4 tsp. orange juice
- 2 tsp. orange peel (zest), grated

Nutrition Per Serving

Calories	133 cal
Protein	24 g
Sodium	97 mg
Phosphorus	214 mg
Dietary Fiber	1.7 g
Potassium	543 mg

Directions
- Preheat the oven to 450° F.
- Mix the celery, carrots, orange zest, and green onions in a small bowl.
- Cut 4 equal parts of the tilapia. Tear off 4 wide foil squares and brush the foil with a nonstick spray.
- Place 1/4 of the vegetables slightly off-center on each sheet of the foil and top with fish. Sprinkle the top of each one with 1 tsp. of orange juice. Use ground black pepper to season.
- To make a pouch or an envelope, fold the foil over it, crimp its edges and place the packets of foil on a baking sheet. Bake for roughly 12 minutes (if the fish is thick, 3-5 minutes longer). Fish, when done, should conveniently split with a fork.
- Remove and put the pouches directly on the plates. When opening, be cautious because of the steam.

33. Mashed Carrots and Ginger

3 servings (1 serving = 1/3 of recipe)

Ingredients
- ½ tsp. fresh chopped ginger
- 2 cups baby carrots
- ½ tsp. Vanilla extract
- ½ tsp. black pepper
- ½ tsp. honey
- Optional garnish: 1 tbsp. chopped fresh chives

Nutrition Per Serving

Calories	30 cal
Protein	1 g
Sodium	55 mg
Phosphorus	21 mg
Dietary Fiber	2 g
Potassium	174 mg

Directions
- At high heat, steam or boil carrots till the carrots are quite tender. Drop heat to low and use a potato masher to mash carrots.
- Add the remaining ingredients (vanilla extract, honey, pepper, and ginger) and stir till well combined.
- **Optional:** Garnish with diced chives and serve.
- **Tip:** Use a blender or food processor for smoother mashed carrots.

34. Aromatic Herbed Rice

6 servings (1 serving = ½ cup)

Ingredients
- 3 cups rice, cooked (but do not overcook)
- 2 tbsp. olive oil
- 2 tbsp. chopped fresh cilantro
- 4–5 sliced thin, cloves fresh garlic
- 2 tbsp. chopped fresh chives
- 2 tbsp. chopped fresh oregano
- 1 tsp. red wine vinegar
- ½ tsp. red pepper flakes

Nutrition Per Serving

Calories	134 cal
Protein	2 g
Sodium	6 mg
Phosphorus	15 mg
Dietary Fiber	1.8 g
Potassium	56 mg

Directions
- Heat the olive oil in a large skillet over medium-high heat and sauté the garlic lightly. Add herbs, flakes of red pepper, and rice and continue cooking for 2-4 minutes or till well-mixed.
- Turn off the flame, mix well and add vinegar.
- Serve

35. Sautéed Collard Greens

6 servings (1 serving = 1/6 portion)

Ingredients
- 2 tbsp. olive oil
- 8 cups fresh, blanched, and chopped collard greens
- ¼ cup finely diced onions
- 1 tsp. ground black pepper
- 1 tbsp. unsalted butter
- 1 tsp. crushed red pepper flakes
- 1 tbsp. chopped fresh garlic
- Optional: 1 tbsp. vinegar

Nutrition Per Serving

Calories	79 cal
Protein	2 g
Sodium	9 mg
Phosphorus	18 mg
Dietary Fiber	2.2 g
Potassium	129 mg

Directions
- Lighten the collard greens by placing them for 30 seconds in a pot of hot water.
- Strain off the boiling water and move the greens to a big bowl of ice water quickly. Let the greens cool off, then strain and dry and put them aside.
- Melt the oil and butter together in a wide sauté pan over medium-high flame. Add the garlic and onions and simmer for around 4-6 minutes, until lightly browned. Add

the collard greens and the red and black pepper, then simmer on high heat for 5-8 minutes, stirring continuously.
- Remove from the heat and, if needed, add vinegar, and stir.

36. Tex Mex Bowl

4 servings (1 serving = 1 Tex Mex Bowl and 10 chips)

Ingredients
- 2 cups canned black beans, low sodium
- 2 cups cooked white quinoa, with 1 tsp. of olive oil
- ½ cup of salsa
- 2 cups shredded iceberg lettuce
- ½ cup regular, cultured sour cream
- 1 cup regular, shredded cheddar cheese
- 40 tortilla corn chips, unsalted
- 4 tbsp. fresh green onion tops

Nutrition Per Serving

Calories	498 kcal
Protein	21 g
Sodium	599 mg
Phosphorus	472 mg
Dietary Fiber	13 g
Potassium	681 mg

Directions
- Rinse, drain, and heat the black beans.
- Into each bowl, layer half a cup of cooked quinoa.
- To each bowl, add half a cup of black beans.
- To each bowl, add half a cup of lettuce.
- Top 2 tbsp. of salsa, 1/4 cup of cheese, 2 tbsp. of sour cream, and 1 tbsp. of green onions to each bowl.
- Serve it with ten tortilla chips.

37. Pasta with a Cheesy Meat Sauce

6 servings (1 serving = 8 oz.)

Ingredients
- 1 lb. ground beef
- ½ box pasta, large-shaped
- 1 tbsp. onion flakes

- ½ cup diced onions
- 1 tbsp. Better Than Bouillon beef (no salt added)
- 1½ cups reduced or no sodium beef stock
- ¾ cup shredded pepper jack or Monterey cheese
- 1 tbsp. tomato sauce (no salt added)
- ½ tsp. Italian seasoning
- 8 oz. softened cream cheese
- 2 tbsp. Reduced sodium, French's Worcestershire sauce
- ½ tsp. ground black pepper

Nutrition Per Serving

Calories	502 cal
Protein	23 g
Sodium	401 mg
Phosphorus	278 mg
Dietary Fiber	1.7 g
Potassium	549 mg

Directions
- As per the instructions on the package, cook pasta noodles.
- Cook the onions, ground beef, and onion flakes in a large skillet till the meat is browned.
- Rinse and add bouillon, tomato sauce, and stock.
- Bring to a boil, occasionally stirring. Stir in the cooked pasta, turn off the heat and add the cream cheese, seasonings (black pepper, Worcestershire sauce, and Italian seasoning) and shredded cheese. Stir in the pasta mixture till all the cheese is melted.
- **Tip:** You may replace ground turkey for beef.

38. Rice Pilaf Baked in Pumpkin

8 servings (2/3 cup each)

Ingredients
- 3 cups cooked rice (made without salt)
- 1 raw pumpkin –3-5 lbs.
- 2 stalks diced celery (or customize with zucchini, peppers, vegetables, or okra)
- 2 small, diced onions
- 2 chopped cloves garlic
- 2 tbsp. canola oil
- 2 diced and peeled carrots
- Fresh herbs of your desire (cilantro, parsley, basil), black pepper or dried herbs

- 1 cup cranberries, dried or fresh

Nutrition Per Serving

Calories	460 cal
Protein	5 g
Sodium	40 mg
Phosphorus	110 mg
Potassium	426 mg

Directions

Both the rice pilaf and pumpkin shell can be cooked ahead of time and kept separately in the fridge till it's time to place it in the oven.

Preparation of Pumpkin Shell
- Cut the top of the pumpkin carefully to make the pumpkin shell. When put back on the pumpkin, just make sure it would fit snugly. Set it aside
- To make the shell empty, clean the inside of the pumpkin. Discard all the seeds and the material inside.
- Place the pumpkin on a baking pan or cookie sheet lined with foil. (Store the pumpkin in the fridge if making ahead.)

Preparation for Filling

Note: You will need to double the rice pilaf ingredients if you've a big pumpkin.
- If not already prepared, prepare the rice to make the pilaf filling. Put it aside.
- In a saucepan, sauté all the vegetables (celery, onions, garlic, carrots) in canola oil till they are tendered.
- Stir in the cranberries, seasonings, and rice.

To Bake
- Preheat the oven to 350°F.
- Spoon the rice pilaf gently into the hollow pumpkin shell and replace the pumpkin top to cover. Put it in a casserole dish if you're not using a pumpkin.
- Bake for almost 60 minutes, or till a fork or knife easily pierces the pumpkin shell. Cover and bake for just 30 minutes or till completely cooked when using a casserole dish.
- Let it cool for 15 minutes at least.
- Serve it warm or at room temperature with a large serving spoon by pulling servings out of the shell.
- To make 8 to 12 wedges, slice through the pumpkin for more fun. Serve the wedge with the pilaf. It'll make the pumpkin tender but firm. Eat just the pumpkin flesh and remove the tough skin.

39. BBQ Ribs with Marinade

16 Servings

Ingredients

- 2 tbsp. brown sugar
- 1/4 cup honey
- 2 tbsp. finely chopped, sweet onion
- 1/4 cup apple cider vinegar
- 1 grated or chopped garlic clove
- 1 cup of water
- 2 tbsp. tomato paste
- 2 tsp. dry mustard
- 1 tbsp. all-purpose flour
- 1 tsp. brown seasoning sauce
- 1 tsp. hot pepper sauce
- 1/4 tsp. Salt
- 1-1/2 tbsp. butter, unsalted

Nutrition Per Serving

Calories	626 cal
Protein	50 g
Sodium	118 mg
Phosphorus	309 mg
Dietary Fiber	0 g
Potassium	490 mg

Directions

BBQ Marinade for the Ribs

- Have the onion finely diced and the garlic clove minced.
- Melt the butter in a saucepan over a low flame.
- Add the garlic and onion and heat till slightly browned.
- Except for the flour, add the rest of the ingredients.
- Continue to heat and stir until mixed, and the sauce continues to simmer lightly over medium flame. Reduce the flame and add flour.
- Whisk till it is mixed and the sauce continues to thicken. Cover the saucepan and set aside for the BBQ grill to marinate the ribs.
- Keep it frozen until you are ready to thaw or use or refrigerate for about 7 days if not used immediately.

Prep Instructions

- Remove the ribs rack from the package. (Scrape off the skin on the back of rack only if the butcher hasn't already done so.)
- Place the ribs rack, with the bottom side up, on the foil.
- Add the marinade to the bottom of the rack, then turn it over.
- Apply some marinade to the rack's top and turn the foil over, covering the top and sides cautiously so that no marinade spills out.
- Save some leftover marinade for the last caramelizing phase on the grill or some for dipping while eating.
- Put your foil coated ribs into the fridge to marinate as you prepare the grill.

40. Shrimp and Coconut Curry Noodle Bowl

5 servings
Ingredients
- 2 tbsp. coconut oil
- 8 oz. rice noodles
- 2 diced summer squash or zucchini
- 1 diced sweet onion
- 2 grated or minced cloves garlic
- 2 corn kernels, ears sweet
- 2-3 tbsp. Thai red curry paste
- 1 tbsp. grated fresh ginger
- 1/3 or 1/2 cup water
- 1 14-oz. full fat, can coconut milk
- 2 tsp. Honey
- 1 tbsp. soy sauce, low sodium
- Top with 1/4 cup cilantro, fresh (or roughly chopped basil)
- Zest and juice from half a lime

Nutrition Per Serving

Calories	418 cal
Protein	16 g
Sodium	195 mg
Phosphorus	285 mg
Dietary Fiber	5 g
Potassium	660 mg

Directions
- As per the instructions given on the package, cook the rice noodles.
- In a broad skillet, heat the coconut oil. Add in it onion and cook over a high flame for at least 5 minutes. Add the corn, zucchini, ginger, and garlic and cook for 5 more minutes till it begins to get soft.

- Mix in the curry paste and simmer for another minute.
- Stir in the water, coconut milk, honey, and soy sauce. Bring it to boil, and simmer till the mixture starts to thicken (for 5 minutes) (about 5 minutes). You may add a little water if the sauce gets too thick.
- Remove the skillet from the flame. Add either the basil or cilantro, according to preference, then whisk in the zest and lime juice.
- Distribute the rice noodles into different bowls for serving and top with a mixture of curry.
- **Optional:** Top with green onions or jalapeño peppers, to taste.

41. Curried Turkey with Rice

6 servings

Ingredients

- 1 lb. turkey breast, sliced into eight cutlets (2 oz.)
- 1 tsp. vegetable oil
- 1 tbsp. margarine, unsalted
- 2 cups white rice, cooked
- 1 chopped, medium onion
- 2 tbsp. Flour
- 1 cup chicken broth, low-sodium
- 2 tsp. curry powder
- 1 tsp. Sugar
- 1/2 cup creamer, non-dairy

Nutrition Per Serving

Calories	154 kcals
Protein	8 g
Sodium	27 mg
Phosphorus	88 mg
Dietary Fiber	1 g
Potassium	156 mg

Directions

- In a broad skillet, heat the oil. Add the turkey and cook, flipping once till no longer pink for at least 10 minutes. Put the turkey on a dish. Wrap in a foil to stay warm.
- In the same skillet, melt the margarine. Add the curry powder and onion. Cook, stirring for at least 5 minutes, then add flour while stirring continuously.
- Stir in sugar, broth, and non-dairy creamer. Stir often till thickened.
- Transfer turkey to the skillet. Cook, flipping to coat till heated through, for approximately 2 minutes.

- Sauce over rice and serve the turkey.

42. Marinated Shrimp

12 servings (serving size 6 shrimp)
Ingredients
- 1 1/2 cup oil
- 2 half lb. large shrimp
- 8 bay leaves
- 2 1/2 tsp. undrained capers
- 3/4 cup white vinegar
- 1 tsp. Salt
- 1 1/2 tsp. celery seeds
- 1 pared, minced garlic clove
- 1 tsp. whole cloves
- 2 cups pared, thinly sliced onions
- Two dashes of sauce or red pepper

Nutrition Per Serving

Calories	188 kcal
Protein	17 g
Sodium	180 mg
Phosphorus	162 mg
Potassium	187 mg

Directions
- Combine all the ingredients mentioned above to make a mixture.
- Take two half lb. large shrimp, which is deveined and cooked in a crab boil. Apply the mixture.
- Alternate the layers of onions, bay leaves, and shrimp mixture in a glass bowl, and place it in a refrigerator for 24 hours. Enjoy.

43. Honey Garlic Chicken

4 servings (serving size: 1/4 roasting chicken that is about 1 lb.)
Ingredients
- 1/2 cup honey
- 4 lb. roasting chicken
- 1 tbsp. olive oil
- 1/2 tsp. black pepper
- 1 tsp. garlic powder

Nutrition Per Serving

Calories	279 kcals
Protein	13 g
Sodium	40 mg
Phosphorus	99 mg
Dietary Fiber	0 g
Potassium	144 mg

Directions

- Preheat the oven to 350 F.
- Grease olive oil on a baking pan.
- Put the chicken in the pan and avoid overlapping pieces. After that, coat the chicken with honey and seasonings.
- Bake for at least 1 hour or till both the sides are brown. During cooking, turn once.

44. Chili Con Carne with Rice

7 servings

Ingredients

- 1 cup onion, chopped
- 1 lb. lean ground beef
- 1 can (6 oz) tomato paste, no-salt-added
- 1 cup green pepper, chopped
- 1 tsp. ground cumin
- 2 tsp. garlic powder
- 1/2 cup pinto beans, cooked (without salt)
- 1 tsp. paprika
- 3-1/2 cups rice, cooked
- 3 cups of water

Nutrition Per Serving

Calories	260 kcals
Protein	15 g
Sodium	63 mg
Phosphorus	144 mg
Dietary Fiber	2 g
Potassium	497 mg

Directions

- In a big pot, brown the ground beef and extract the fat.
- Add the green pepper and onion and cook till the onion becomes transparent. Add the rest of the ingredients and cook for 1-1/2 hours.

- Serve over scalding hot rice.

45. Honey Mustard Sauce and Chicken Nuggets

12 servings (serving size: 3 nuggets with 1 tbsp. sauce)
Ingredients
- 1 tbsp. Dijon mustard
- 1 lb. chicken breast, boneless, sliced into 36 pieces (bite-sized)
- 1/3 cup honey
- 1/2 cup mayonnaise
- Nonstick cooking spray
- 1 beaten egg
- 2 tsp. Worcestershire sauce
- 3 cups low sodium cornflakes, finely crushed
- 2 tbsp. non-dairy creamer, liquid

Nutrition Per Serving

Calories	166 kcals
Protein	7 g
Sodium	184 mg
Phosphorus	67 mg
Dietary Fiber	0.5 g
Potassium	99 mg

Directions
- Stir mayonnaise, Worcestershire sauce, honey, and mustard together in a tiny bowl. Chill sauce till nuggets are ready, after which serve as a dipping sauce.
- Preheat the oven to 400°F.
- Combine the non-dairy creamer and egg in a medium bowl. Crush the cornflakes and place them into a big zip-lock bag.
- Dip the chicken pieces in the mixture of egg, then dip in a zip-lock bag to cover with the cornflake crumbs.
- On a baking sheet coated with non-stick cooking spray, bake the nuggets for 15 minutes or till they are done.

46. Chicken Enchiladas

7 servings
Ingredients
Enchilada Sauce:
- 2 minced cloves garlic

- 1 tbsp. olive oil
- 1/2 tsp. oregano, dried
- 1 tsp. onion, minced
- 1/2 tsp. basil, dried
- 1 cup of water
- 2 1/2 tsp. chili powder
- 1/2 tsp. ground cumin
- 1/2 tsp. ground black pepper
- 6-oz. can tomato sauce, no-salt
- 2 tsp. minced parsley

Enchiladas:
- 2 tbsp. canola oil
- 8 oz. shredded, boiled chicken (2 chicken breasts)
- 7 oz. can green chiles, diced
- 1 cup Monterey jack cheese, shredded
- 1 chopped, medium onion
- 8 oz. sour cream
- 8 oz. chicken broth, low sodium
- 6"- flour tortillas
- 3 chopped green onions

Nutrition Per Serving

Calories	351 kcals
Protein	17 g
Sodium	347 mg
Phosphorus	238 mg
Dietary Fiber	3 g
Potassium	474 mg

Directions
Enchilada Sauce:
- Heat the oil over medium flame in a saucepan. Add the onion and garlic and sauté for at least 2 minutes.
- Add the remaining ingredients and boil them. Low the flame and simmer for 15-20 minutes. Set it aside.

Enchiladas:
- Preheat the oven to 350 F.
- Heat the oil over medium flame in a large skillet. Add the onions, then cook for 5 minutes.

- Mix in the green chili peppers, chicken broth, and chicken. Bring to the boil, reduce the flame, and cook for 15 minutes.
- Combine half of the green onions and sour cream.
- Spoon the 1/3-cup mixture of chicken onto each tortilla. Roll the tortilla up and put the seam in a 9-9 baking dish in a single layer. Garnish with the cheese, enchilada sauce, and leftover green onion.
- For 30 minutes, bake.

47. Garlic Shrimp

5 servings

Ingredients
- 1 cup melted margarine, unsalted
- 1 lb. Shrimp in shells
- 1 clove garlic, minced
- 1/8 tsp. pepper
- 2 tsp. lemon juice
- 1 tbsp. fresh parsley, chopped
- 2 tbsp. onion, chopped

Nutrition Per Serving

Calories	404 kcals
Protein	14 g
Sodium	105 mg
Phosphorus	157 mg
Dietary Fiber	0 g
Potassium	153 mg

Directions
- Preheat the broiler.
- Wash the shrimp and dry it.
- Add the margarine, onion, lemon juice, pepper, and garlic to a shallow baking pan.
- Add the shrimp and flip to coat.
- For 5 minutes, broil. For 5 more minutes, turn and broil.
- Serve with strained pan juices on a platter. With parsley, sprinkle.
- Peel the shrimp and eat.

48. Beef Ribs

Serves about 8 ribs

Ingredients
- 1/4 cup of pineapple juice
- 4 lb. beef ribs, large
- 1/8 tsp. red pepper
- 2 tsp. chili powder
- 1 tbsp. paprika
- 1/2 tsp. garlic powder
- 1/4 tsp. mustard powder

Nutrition Per Serving

Calories	187 kcals
Protein	19 g
Sodium	41 mg
Phosphorus	149 mg
Dietary Fiber	0 g
Potassium	233 mg

Directions
- Put a single layer of ribs in 2 shallow roastings pans, with meat side down on the racks. Roast for 30 minutes in a 450 degrees F oven. Drain.
- Brush the ribs with the juice of pineapple.
- Mix the rest of the ingredients together. Sprinkle uniformly on the ribs.
- Lower the oven to 350 degrees F. Roast the ribs for another 45 to 60 minutes with the meaty side up.

49. Sukiyaki and Rice

10 servings

Ingredients
- 1 tbsp. vegetable oil
- 2 1/2 lb. lean beef chuck (slice into thin paper pieces)
- 1/2 cup celery (diced into 1/2-inch slices)
- 1 cup white turnip (diced into 1/8-inch pieces)
- 3 scallions (sliced thin), medium
- 1 green pepper, medium (diced in rings)
- 1 onion, medium (dice into 1/8-inch pieces)
- 1 cup cabbage, shredded
- 3/4 cup mushrooms, sliced
- 1 tomato, medium size, sliced
- 1/2 cup broccoli, chopped and frozen
- 1 tbsp. Sugar

- 2 tbsp. soy sauce, low sodium
- 5 cups white rice, cooked
- 1 tbsp. Water

Nutrition Per Serving

Calories	495 kcals
Protein	24 g
Sodium	161 mg
Phosphorus	251 mg
Dietary Fiber	2 g
Potassium	536 mg

Directions
- Put the oil in a big heavy skillet (mostly electric is suitable), on both sides, lightly brown meat.
- Turn the heat to simmer and add the vegetables into the skillet (in layers).
- Combine the sugar, water, and soy sauce, and spill over the vegetables.
- Cover and steam for 10-15 minutes under the moderate flame. Don't stir.
- Serve with simmering rice (per serving, half cup rice.

50. Spicy Pork Chops with Apples

6 servings (serving size: 1 chop)

Ingredients
- 3/4 tsp. of salt
- 2 minced Garlic cloves, pared
- 1 red onion, large and pared, sliced into 3/4-inch slices
- 1/2 tsp. of sugar
- 1.2 tsp. of ground ginger
- 1/4 tsp. of ground cumin
- 1/4 tsp. of pepper
- 2 unpaired, medium, cored Rome Beauty apples, diced into 1-inch slices
- 6 pork chops, large

Nutrition Per Serving

Calories	215 kcals
Protein	15 g
Sodium	330 mg
Phosphorus	126 mg
Potassium	288 mg

Directions

- Combine the garlic cloves, salt, ground ginger, sugar, pepper, and ground cumin.
- Rub the seasoning mixture onto each pork chop on both sides.
- Put it in a wide glass pan.
- Between the chops, insert slices of onions and apples.
- Crumple the aluminum foil and put it at every end of the pan in order to press together the ingredients.
- Cover with the foil and bake for 20 minutes at 400F.
- Lower the heat to 325F and bake for 30-35 minutes.
- Uncover.
- To separate the chops, extract the crumpled foil; and bake for approximately 15 minutes till light brown.
- Serve over rice.

51. Shrimp Scampi

6 servings

Ingredients

- 5 chopped cloves garlic
- 1 1/2 lb. Shrimp
- 1/2 cup of white wine
- 1/2 cup of butter

Nutrition Per Serving

Calories	265 kcals
Protein	24 g
Sodium	412 mg
Phosphorus	166 mg
Dietary Fiber	0 g
Potassium	238 mg

Directions

- Peel the Shrimp.
- In butter, sauté garlic.
- Add the shrimp and simmer till barely white.
- Add the wine to prepare and cook (at least 3 to 5 minutes).
- Serve with rice or pasta

52. Rosemary Chicken

4 servings
Ingredients
- 1/3 cup of brown sugar
- 1 broiler-fryer chicken, split in half or sliced into quarters
- 1/2 cup white wine, dry
- 1/4 cup lime juice
- 1/4 cup oil such as safflower, sunflower, or canola
- 1 tsp. Worcestershire sauce
- 2 tsp. dried, crushed rosemary

Nutrition Per Serving

Calories	539 kcals
Protein	36.5 g
Sodium	136 mg
Phosphorus	254 mg
Dietary Fiber	0.4 g
Potassium	412 mg

Directions
- Combine all the ingredients, excluding chicken, in a shallow dish to render marinade.
- Add the chicken and flip to cover with marinade. Cover it and refrigerate for at least 3-4 hours, flipping occasionally.
- Drain the chicken, reserving marinade for the basting.
- Put the chicken, with the skin side down, on the rack in a broiling pan, about 7 - 9 inches from the source of heat. Broil for at least 20 minutes, sometimes basting the chicken with marinade. Turn it, dust gently with marinade, then broil 15 minutes further or till fork tender.
- Discard the leftover marinade.

53. Rock Cornish Game Hens and Tarragon

4 servings (serving size 1/2 hen)
Ingredients
- 1 sliced, pared garlic clove
- 2 Rock Cornish (1 1/4 lb. each) Game hens, split
- 1/4 lb. Margarine
- Ground pepper (as needed), fresh.
- 1 tbsp. chopped fresh parsley.
- 1 tbsp. Tarragon

Nutrition Per Serving

Calories	286 cal
Protein	24 g
Sodium	71 mg
Phosphorus	160 mg
Potassium	235 mg

Directions

- Trim extra fat from the tail and skin from the neck. Rub the skin with garlic, gently dust with pepper. Place the hens, with the skin side up, in a 2-inch-deep baking pan.
- Heat margarine till melted, add parsley and tarragon; mix thoroughly. Bake the hens at 350F, whisking with a mixture of tarragon every 15 minutes for an hour. Drain off the margarine before serving.

54. Red Pepper Roasted Pesto

2 servings

Ingredients

- 1 jar (about 7-8 oz.) red bell peppers, roasted, drained.
- 2 garlic cloves (diced in half)
- ¼ cup tor, fresh basil
- ¼ cup olive oil
- pepper to taste
- 1 tsp. balsamic vinegar
- meat-filled tortellini or ravioli.

Nutrition Per Serving

Calories	526 kcals
Protein	17 g
Sodium	487 mg
Phosphorus	186 mg
Dietary Fiber	2 g
Potassium	394 mg

Directions

- In a food processor, mix all the ingredients, excluding the pasta and blend for 30 seconds until it achieves perfect consistency. Taste, and modify tastes to your liking.
- As per the guidance on the packet, cook the stuffed pasta or ravioli. Don't salt the pasta water; the ravioli and sauce contain a lot of sodium.
- Cover the hot ravioli with pesto instantly and enjoy.

55. Alaska Baked Macaroni with Cheese

8 SERVINGS

Ingredients
- 2 tbsp. flour
- 3 cups small shell, elbow, or bowtie pasta
- 2 cups milk
- chopped almonds or croutons to taste.
- 2 tbsp. butter, unsalted
- 1 tsp. paprika
- 1 tsp. mustard powder
- 2 cups cheese (cheddar, gouda, or any combo)
- 1 tbsp. Tarragon or fresh thyme chopped or 1 tsp. dry.

Nutrition Per Serving

Calories	424 cal
Protein	22 g
Sodium	479 mg
Phosphorus	428 mg
Dietary Fiber	2 g
Potassium	237 mg

Directions
- Heat the oven to 350 degrees F.
- Boil the pasta in a wide pot till al-dente.
- In a glass (medium size) measuring cup, weigh butter and flour. Microwave between 1-2 minutes till golden brown.
- Gently stir in the milk and keep microwaving till thickened. Stir in herbs and spices.
- Mix sauce, drained noodles, and cheese and place in an oiled casserole dish. Bake for 20 minutes.
- Cover with chopped almonds or croutons in the last 5 minutes.

56. Baked Potato Soup

6 SERVINGS (1 1/2 CUP EACH)

Ingredients
- 1/3 cup flour
- 2 potatoes, large
- 1/2 tsp. pepper
- 4 cups skim milk
- 1/2 cup sour cream, fat-free
- 4 oz. reduce fat, shredded Monterey jack cheese.

Nutrition Per Serving

Calories	216 cal
Protein	15 g
Sodium	272 mg
Phosphorus	326 mg
Dietary Fiber	4 g
Potassium	594 mg

Directions
- At 400 F, bake the potatoes till the fork-tender.
- Let it cool.
- Slice it lengthwise and scoop the pulp out.
- Put the flour in a big saucepan. Add the milk gradually, mixing till blended.
- Add pepper and potato pulp.
- Cook it till bubbly and thick, over medium heat, mixing frequently.
- Add the cheese and stir till it melts.
- Remove from the flame and mix in the sour cream.

57. Chicken or Beef Enchiladas

6 servings

Ingredients
- 1/2 cup chopped onion.
- 1 can enchilada sauce
- 1 lb. lean ground chicken or beef
- 1/2 tsp. black pepper
- 1 tsp. cumin
- 12 corn tortillas
- 1 chopped garlic clove

Nutrition Per Serving

Calories	235 cal
Protein	13 g
Sodium	201 mg
Phosphorus	146 mg
Dietary Fiber	14 g
Potassium	222 mg

Directions
- Preheat the oven to 375°F.
- Brown the meat in a saucepan.

- Add the garlic, onion, pepper, and cumin. Keep cooking. Stir till you have soft onions.
- Fry the tortillas in another pan in a small quantity of oil.
- In an enchilada sauce, dip each tortilla.
- Fill with the mixture of meat and roll them up.
- In a shallow pan, put the enchilada and, if desired, cover it with cheese and sauce.
- Bake until the enchiladas are golden brown, and the cheese is melted
- Serve with your choice of sliced olives, sour cream, or some other topping.

58. Broccoli Chicken Casserole

6 SERVINGS

Ingredients
- 1 chopped, medium onion
- 2-3 cups of cooked broccoli
- grated parmesan for topping
- 2 tbsp. margarine or butter
- 2-3 diced chicken breast
- 2 cups milk
- 2 beaten eggs
- 2 cups cheese, grated
- 2 cups cooked barley, noodles, or rice

Nutrition Per Serving

Calories	368 cal
Protein	26 g
Sodium	388 mg
Phosphorus	243 mg
Potassium	371 mg

Directions
- Preheat the oven to 350°F.
- Put the broccoli in a microwaveable dish, cover it with plastic wrap, and microwave for almost 2-3 minutes till bright green.
- In the meanwhile, brown chicken, and onion in the butter in the skillet.
- Combine all the ingredients in an oiled casserole dish and mix.
- Sprinkle the top with the grated parmesan cheese and bake for at least 1 hour and 15 minutes, till set and the fork comes out clean.

59. Chicken' N Corn Chowder

12 SERVINGS

Ingredients
- 2 chopped onions
- 12 slices low sodium bacon
- 4 soaked and diced potatoes
- 7 cups low sodium, chicken broth
- 8 chicken breasts, boneless and diced
- 8 cups Corn
- 4 cups Mocha Mix
- 6 tbsp. chopped, fresh thyme
- 8 chopped green onions
- 1/2 tsp. black pepper

Nutrition Per Serving

Calories	472 cal
Protein	31 g
Sodium	260 mg
Phosphorus	438 mg
Dietary Fiber	15 g
Potassium	1172 mg

Directions
- Cook the bacon in a skillet till crisp, remove the bacon and put aside.
- Sauté the onions in the bacon fat.
- Add the potatoes and broth.
- Cover and cook for 10 mins.
- Add chicken, thyme, and corn.
- Cover and cook till the chicken is cooked for at least 15 mins.
- Stir the Mocha, mix into the soup and cook for 2 minutes.
- Sprinkle in pepper, green onions, and bacon.

60. Chicken and Dumplings

8 SERVINGS

Ingredients
- 2 cups water or chicken broth, low sodium
- 3 lbs. chopped chicken or 1 whole chicken
- 2-3 sliced carrots
- 1 stalk celery with leaves (cut fine)
- 1/2 tsp. mace or nutmeg
- 1/2 tsp. black pepper
- 2 eggs
- 1/4 cup flour

- 3 tsp. baking powder
- 2/3 cup milk
- 2 tbsp. margarine or unsalted butter
- 2 cups flour

Nutrition Per Serving

Calories	401 cal
Protein	45 g
Sodium	146 mg
Phosphorus	584 mg
Dietary Fiber	2 g
Potassium	940 mg

Directions
- In a slow cooker, add vegetables, water or broth, spices, and chicken.
- Pour more water that is enough to cover around 1" chicken.
- Turn the cooker to low flame for 6-8 hours.
- Remove the chicken to a dish that is ovenproof.
- If you like, remove the bones. They might just fall off.
- Cover it and keep warm.
- Turn the slow cooker to maximum heat. To prevent lumps, add 1/4 cup flour and stir rapidly.
- Slice the butter using two knives, a food processor, or a pastry cutter, into the two flour cups.
- Mix in wet ingredients to a dough and spill into the boiling broth with a spoonful.
- Cap the cooker, reduce the flame to avoid boiling and cook without removing the lid for 15 minutes.
- Serve with the dumplings, place the chicken in a large serving dish, and spill thickened sauce over it.

61. Chicken Seafood Gumbo

12, one-cup servings

Ingredients
- 3 chopped celery stalks
- 1 tbsp. canola oil
- 1 chopped, red bell pepper
- 1 chopped yellow onion
- 8 oz. sliced, lean smoked turkey sausage
- 3 cups chopped, frozen okra
- 2 skinless, chopped chicken breasts

- 1/2 cup flour
- 1/2 cup canola oil
- 2 quarts chicken broth, low sodium
- 1 tbsp. Cajun seasoning, salt-free
- 6 oz. drained, canned crab
- 1/2 lb. cooked shrimp

Nutrition Per Serving

Calories	240 cal
Protein	10 g
Sodium	320 mg
Phosphorus	156 mg
Dietary Fiber	14 g
Potassium	426 mg

Directions

- In a 4.5-quart or larger pot, over medium flame, heat 1 tbsp. of canola oil.
- Cook for at least 10 minutes and add onion, celery, bell pepper, sausage, and chicken.
- Set it aside while removing the mixture from the pot.
- Reduce the flame to medium.
- To make a roux, add 1/2 cup of canola oil and whisk in the flour.
- Mix in Cajun seasoning, based on how dark you like your gumbo to be, then let it simmer for one minute or more.
- Stir in the chicken broth very slowly, stir continuously to prevent lumps.
- Bring the mixture to a boil and boil for at least 10 minutes or till it begins to thicken gradually. Raise the flame to medium-high.
- Reduce the flame to medium, add the crab, shrimp, and okra, and return the chicken mixture to the pot.
- Cook for at least 10 minutes or till fully heated.

62. Chicken and Cornbread Stuffing

4 servings

Ingredients

- 2 tbsp. + 1 1/2 tsp. divided, Mrs. Dash Original Blend
- 1 tbsp. fresh parsley
- 4 (4 oz.) pieces skinless, boneless, chicken breast halves
- 1 cup chicken broth, low sodium, fat-free
- 1 tbsp. Chicken Grilling Blend (Mrs. Dash)
- 1 cup chopped celery

- 1 tbsp. unsalted butter
- 2 tsp. ground sage
- 1/2 cup chopped onion
- 2 cups croutons, unseasoned
- 2 cups (7 oz.) coarsely crumbled cornbread

Nutrition Per Serving

Calories	372 cal
Protein	28 g
Sodium	478 mg
Phosphorus	204 mg
Potassium	414 mg

Directions
- Chop the parsley.
- Combine 1 tbsp. of Mrs. Dash Original Blend with Chicken Grilling Blend, and parsley. Mix lightly.
- Coat the chicken breasts with seasoning mixture on both sides.
- Spray with cooking spray (non-stick) on a large non-stick skillet.
- Heat the skillet till hot, over medium flame.
- Add the chicken breasts to the skillet and cook on each side for 3 to 5 minutes till light brown.
- Set aside while removing the chicken breasts from the skillet.
- Preheat the oven to 350°F.
- Melt the butter over a low flame in a skillet.
- Add 1 tbsp. + 1 1/2 tsp. of Mrs. Dash Original Blend, onion, and celery, sage, combine to blend.
- Cook for 5 to 7 minutes over medium flame or till the vegetables is soft.
- Remove from the flame.
- In a mixing bowl, combine the croutons and cornbread crumbs.
- Add the mixture of vegetables and the broth, then combine to blend.
- Spoon the dressing mixture on a baking dish, gently brushed with a non-stick cooking spray.
- Arrange the chicken breasts on the top of the dressing mixture.
- Wrap and bake for 45 minutes at 350 F.
- Continue to bake for 5 to 10 minutes or till the chicken breast has an internal temperature of 170°.
- Garnish, if needed, with celery leaves.

63. Chinese Chicken Salad

8 servings

Ingredients

- 3 tbsp. olive oil, divided
- 2 packages noodles, ramen
- 1/2 cup rice vinegar or white wine vinegar
- 2 cups cooked, diced turkey or chicken
- 2 tbsp. sesame seeds
- 4 diced green onions
- 1/2 head chopped and shredded cabbage
- 1 tbsp. sesame oil
- 1/4 cup Splenda or sugar

Nutrition Per Serving

Calories	203 cal
Protein	19 g
Sodium	48 mg
Phosphorus	41 mg
Potassium	259 mg

Directions

- Take the noodles and crush them while they are still in the packet.
- Open the packs and remove the packs of seasoning.
- In a skillet, heat 1 tbsp. of olive oil.
- Add the sesame seeds and dry noodles.
- Toast till golden brown.
- In a bowl, mix the turkey or chicken, green onions, and cabbage, then add the sesame seeds and ramen noodles.
- In a separate bowl, combine the sugar, 2 tbsp. of olive oil, vinegar, and sesame oil.
- Place the dressing in the salad.

64. Cider Cream Chicken

8 servings

Ingredients

- 2 tbsp. butter, unsalted
- 4 chicken breasts, bone-in
- 1/2 cup half and half
- 3/4 cup of apple cider

Nutrition Per Serving

Calories	186 cal
Protein	27 g
Sodium	83 mg
Phosphorus	266 mg
Potassium	414 mg

Directions
- Melt the butter over the high-medium flame. Add the chicken and brown both sides.
- Add the cider and lower the flame to medium; cook for almost 20 minutes to simmer.
- Remove the chicken from the skillet.
- Boil the cider till decreased to at least 1/4 cup.
- Overheat, add half and half; whisk till thickened slightly.
- Pour the cream sauce over the chicken and enjoy.

65. Confetti Chicken and Rice

4 servings

Ingredients
- 1 skinless, boneless chicken breast
- 3 tbsp. divided olive oil
- 1 fresh, cubed zucchini
- 3 ears, kernels extracted or 2 1/4 cups frozen corn, no salt added
- 1 medium, diced red onion
- 1 large, cubed red bell pepper
- 1 tbsp. cumin
- 1/2 tsp. garlic powder
- 2 tsp. Mrs. Dash original
- 1/2 tsp. black pepper
- 1 package original ready rice, Uncle Ben's
- 1/4 tsp. cayenne pepper

Nutrition Per Serving

Calories	519 cal
Protein	17 g
Sodium	37 mg
Phosphorus	152 mg
Dietary Fiber	14 g
Potassium	316 mg

Directions

- Heat 2 tbsp. of olive oil in a large non-stick skillet over medium-high flame.
- Put the chicken breast wisely in the skillet when the oil is hot.
- Remove the chicken from the skillet once the juices are clear (about 15 minutes)
- Add 1 tbsp. of olive oil, zucchini, corn, onion, and red pepper to the same skillet.
- Sauté till the onions start caramelizing on medium to medium-high flame. (about 10 minutes).
- Then add the cumin, garlic powder, black pepper, cayenne pepper and Mrs. Dash.
- Cube the chicken and return to pan with vegetables, lower the flame to medium-low and continue the mixture stirring for 5 minutes or so.
- Follow the rice package instructions.
- Add to the vegetables when the rice is ready and proceed to sauté for a couple more minutes.
- Enjoy!

66. Crab Cakes and Lime Ginger Sauce

8 servings

Ingredients
- 1/2 cup finely diced onion
- 1/2 cup finely diced celery
- 3 cups well-drained crab meat
- 1 medium, finely diced red bell pepper
- 1 cup mayonnaise
- 2 eggs
- 1 tsp. Worcestershire sauce
- 1/2 cup lemon juice
- 1 tbsp. minced chives
- 1/2 tsp. hot pepper sauce
- 1 tsp. minced fresh garlic
- 1 tsp. minced fresh thyme
- 1 recipe ginger sauce, lime
- 3/4 cup of panko crumbs

Nutrition Per Serving

Calories	354 cal
Protein	12 g
Sodium	444 mg
Phosphorus	133 mg
Potassium	279 mg

Directions
- Fold all the ingredients except for the panko together gently in a wide bowl.
- Sprinkle some panko gently on a baking sheet.
- With an ice cream scoop, scoop out mounds of a mixture of crab and put them on the baking sheet.
- One by one, in panko, dredge mounds, shaping into the cakes while you go.
- Wrap and refrigerate.
- On a medium-high flame, heat some oil in a skillet.
- Add the crab cakes and sauté for 4 minutes per side, till they are golden brown.
- Remove the paper towels and rinse.
- Per recipe, make Lime Ginger Sauce and place it on the side.

67. Creamy Tuna Twist

4-1 cup servings

Ingredients
- 2 tbsp. vinegar
- 3/4 cup mayonnaise
- 1 tbsp. dried dill weed
- 1 can (6 1/2 oz.) tuna, drained, water-packed, or unsalted
- 1 1/2 cups cooked, shell macaroni
- 1/2 cup (chopped pea size) celery
- 1/2 cup cooked peas

Nutrition Per Serving

Calories	421 cal
Protein	15 g
Sodium	379 mg
Phosphorus	122 mg
Potassium	204 mg

Directions
- In a large bowl, stir together the vinegar, mayonnaise, and macaroni shells till smooth.
- Add the remaining ingredients, then stir until mixed.
- Cover and chill.

68. Chili Verde, Crock Pot

6-8 servings

Ingredients
- 2 large onions (sliced into wedges)
- 2-2 1/2 lbs. pork loin chops or pork, trim fat
- 1 red bell pepper sliced into 1-inch squares
- 1 1/2 tbsp. corn starch
- 2 cups tomatillos, fresh or 1 jar (16 oz.) Green Tomatillo Salsa and 1/2 cup vinegar
- 3/4 tsp. garlic powder
- 1/2 cup beef broth, low-sodium
- 1 green bell pepper sliced into 1-inch squares
- 1/2-3/4 tsp. red chili flakes

Nutrition Per Serving

Calories	227 cal
Protein	6 g
Sodium	43 mg
Phosphorus	83 mg
Dietary Fiber	13 g
Potassium	222 mg

Directions
- In a slow cooker of 3 1/2-4 quarts. Layer chops of pork, tomatillos or sauce of green tomatillo and onions.
- Mix the cornstarch into the broth, add the vinegar (only if you are using fresh tomatillos), red chili flakes, and garlic powder to the crockpot.
- Wrap and cook on low heat for 6 1/2-7 hours or until tender.
- Raise the heat to a high setting.
- Stir in the bell peppers, both green and red.
- Cover and simmer for 15 minutes to half an hour on high.
- Pour over the corn chips with low salt or serve with the rice.

69. Crock Pot Chicken Chili White

12-14 servings
Ingredients
- 1 cup black-eyed peas, dried
- 1 cup Great Northern beans, dried
- 1/2 cup small lima beans, dried
- 1 cup lima beans, dried
- 2 diced, medium onions
- 8 cups water
- 2 lbs. diced chicken breast

- 3 tbsp. garlic, minced
- 2 tbsp. canola or vegetable oil
- 1-2 diced jalapeño chili peppers
- 2 tsp. cumin
- 2 cups corn, frozen
- 1 tsp. black pepper
- 2 tsp. oregano
- 2 cups sour cream
- 1/2 tsp. cayenne pepper

Nutrition Per Serving

Calories	306 cal
Protein	25 g
Sodium	75 mg
Phosphorus	321 mg
Dietary Fiber	9 g
Potassium	845 mg

Directions
- Rinse the dried beans and sort them out.
- Put the beans with water in the crockpot / slow cooker.
- Set a low temperature.
- Meanwhile, sauté the onions, diced chicken, jalapeños, and garlic in canola oil or vegetables in a skillet, for at least 10 minutes, till lightly browned.
- Add it to the Crock-Pot.
- To the mixture, add spices and corn.
- Allow 9-11 hours to cook, or overnight.
- Mix in the sour cream before serving.

70. Dijon Chicken

4 servings

Ingredients
- 1/4 cup of Dijon mustard
- 1 tsp. curry powder
- 4 chicken breasts, boneless
- 1 tsp. lemon Juice
- 3 tbsp. honey

Nutrition Per Serving

Calories	189 cal
Protein	25 g

Sodium	258 mg
Phosphorus	250 mg
Dietary Fiber	3 g
Potassium	454 mg

Directions

- Preheat the oven to 350°F.
- In a baking dish, place the chicken.
- In a bowl, mix the other ingredients.
- Brush the chicken with sauce on both sides.
- Bake for at least 30 minutes or till the internal temperature of the chicken reaches 165 degrees F.

71. Dilled Fish

6 servings

Ingredients

- 1 tsp. instant, minced (freeze-dried) onion
- 1 1/2 lbs. firm white fish, fresh
- 1/2 tsp. dill weed
- 1/4 tsp. mustard powder
- 4 tsp. lemon Juice
- A dash of pepper

Nutrition Per Serving

Calories	112 cal
Protein	23 g
Sodium	63 mg
Phosphorus	194 mg
Potassium	350 mg

Directions

- Preheat the oven to 475°F.
- Rinse the fish and dry it.
- Place it in a baking dish.
- Combine 2 tbsp. of water with mustard, onion, pepper, and dill weed.
- To spice it, add lemon Juice and spill evenly over the fish.
- Bake for 17-20 minutes, uncovered.

72. Fast Fajitas

4 (two fajitas each) servings

Ingredients
- Zest of lime or 1 lime juice
- 1 tbsp. olive oil
- 1 tsp. cumin
- Zest of orange or lemon and 1 lemon juice
- cilantro to taste
- 1 lb. shrimp, meat, tofu, bite-size pieces
- Dash cayenne pepper
- 2 sliced bell peppers
- 1 sliced onion
- sour cream (according to taste)
- 8 corn tortillas

Nutrition Per Serving

Calories	320 cal
Protein	29 g
Sodium	142 mg
Phosphorus	332 mg
Dietary Fiber	8 g
Potassium	445 mg

Directions
- In a small bowl, combine the citrus zest, oil, cumin, cayenne pepper, and Juice to create the marinade. Place in a shallow dish or a bag the vegetables, marinade, and meat, and marinate overnight.
- Cook the marinated vegetables and meat in a large skillet on medium flame till the onions start to caramelize or turn light brown and soft and meat is cooked through. This is supposed to take 15-20 minutes at least.
- Serve with tortillas and also top with cilantro and sour cream.

73. Fast Roast Chicken with Herbs & Lemon

4-6 (three oz. servings) servings

Ingredients
- 2 tbsp. butter, softened and unsalted
- 1 (4-5 oz.) fresh or thawed whole chicken
- 2 crushed and peeled cloves garlic
- 2 1/2 tbsp. fresh herbs (thyme, sage etc.), chopped
- 1 tbsp. olive oil
- 1 small, thinly sliced lemon

Nutrition Per Serving

Calories	251 cal
Protein	19 g
Sodium	77 mg
Phosphorus	188 mg
Dietary Fiber	18 g
Potassium	222 mg

Directions

- Preheat the oven to 450°F.
- In a roasting pan, put the chicken in it.
- In a little bowl, combine the herbs, garlic, and butter.
- Put the herbed butter together with the lemon slices within the chicken's body cavity.
- Apply the olive oil over the bird's skin.
- Roast for at least 15 minutes per pound or till the temperature exceeds 165 degrees F.
- Drain the lemon slices and the buttery juices and spill over the chicken.
- Before slicing, let the chicken rest for almost 20 minutes.

74. Fresh Marinara Sauce

16 servings

Ingredients

- 1 pot water, boiling
- 6 lbs. or 15 medium tomatoes, ripe or 2- 28 oz. cans tomatoes, low sodium
- 2 large, chopped onions
- 6 minced garlic cloves
- 1/3 cup olive oil
- 1 tsp. pepper
- 3-4 large, grated carrots
- 1 tbsp. Dry or 3 tbsp. oregano, fresh
- 1/3 cup chopped, fresh basil or 2 tbsp. dry

Nutrition Per Serving

Calories	80 cal
Protein	2 g
Sodium	25 mg
Phosphorus	46 mg
Potassium	341 mg

Directions

- If you are using fresh tomatoes, add a few to the boiling water at a time and cover for at least 1 minute.
- Use a slotted spoon to lift them out and put them into cold water.
- To get 11 to 12 cups, strip off the skin and coarsely cut the tomatoes.
- Chop coarsely when using canned tomatoes, low sodium.
- Cook the onion, carrots, and garlic in medium-hot oil in a 5-quart or broader kettle, occasionally stirring, till the onions are translucent.
- Add the tomatoes, pepper, basil, and oregano.
- Bring to a boil, minimize heat, and cook steadily, uncovered, and frequently stirring until the sauce is thickened. Serve over the pasta
- Until needed, freeze the extra sauce in food storage bags or freezer containers.

75. Fruit Vinegar Chicken

6 servings

Ingredients
- 1/2 cup berry or fruit vinegar
- 2 lbs. chicken
- 1/2 tsp. tarragon
- 1/4 cup orange Juice
- 1/4 cup oil
- 1/2 tsp. basil
- 1/2 tsp. marjoram

Nutrition Per Serving

Calories	413 cal
Protein	28 g
Sodium	106 mg
Phosphorus	227 mg
Potassium	335 mg

Directions
- Preheat the oven to 350°F.
- Combine in a big zip lock bag all the ingredients.
- 15-20 minutes marinade in the refrigerator.
- Take the chicken out of the bag and place it in a baking dish.
- Bake for approximately 30 minutes or till the internal temperature of the chicken exceeds 165 degrees F.

76. Fruity Chicken Salad

8 servings

Ingredients
- 1 cup almonds, sliced
- 2 cups cubed or cooked chicken breasts, and or 12.5 oz. chicken, canned
- 1 chopped green onion
- 1 chopped stalk celery
- 1 cubed apple
- 2 cups grapes, seedless
- 1/2 cup sour cream
- 3/4 cup raisins
- 1 tsp. unseasoned rice vinegar
- 1/4 cup mayo
- 1/2 tsp. Chinese Five-Spice Blend
- 2 tsp. sugar

Nutrition Per Serving

Calories	279 cal
Protein	15 g
Sodium	82 mg
Phosphorus	159 mg
Potassium	352 mg

Directions
- Combine the almonds, chicken, celery, grapes, green onion, raisins, and apples in a large bowl.
- Combine the sour cream, rice vinegar, mayo, Chinese Five-Spice Blend, and sugar in a separate bowl.
- Mix the dressing in the chicken mixture.

77. Grilled Lemon Kebabs (Chicken)

2 servings

Ingredients
- 2 lemons
- 4 pieces skinless, boneless chicken thighs
- 1 crushed and peeled clove garlic
- 1 tsp. white wine vinegar
- 3 tbsp. olive oil
- 2 bay leaves (torn in half)
- 1 tbsp. fresh herbs (thyme, sage etc.), chopped

Nutrition Per Serving

Calories	362 cal
Protein	27 g
Sodium	119 mg
Phosphorus	238 mg
Dietary Fiber	25 g
Potassium	404 mg

Directions
- Each thigh is chopped into chunky pieces and put in a bowl.
- Grate 1 tsp. of lemon zest and Juice the leftover lemon.
- Add the oil, herbs, vinegar, and garlic to the chicken.
- For at least 3 hours or overnight, cover and marinate.
- Slice four thick slices of the other lemon, then cut up each slice into four pieces.
- Alternate the chicken pieces and lemon slices on a wooden skewer, pack as tight as possible and finish with a piece of lemon.
- For each skewer, repeat.
- Grill in the oven, countertop-type grill, or barbecue till done, approximately 10 minutes on each side.

78. Honey Herb Glazed Turkey

6-8 servings

Ingredients
- 1 onion, sliced into wedges
- 10-12 lbs. whole turkey
- 1 lemon, sliced into chunks
- 2 whole celery stalks
- 1/2 cup butter, unsalted
- 1/3 cup olive oil
- 1/3 cup thyme, freshly stripped from stems (14 stems)
- 2 tbsp. sage leaves, fresh
- 2 tsp. celery seed
- 2 bay leaves, fresh
- 2 tsp. lemon Juice
- 1/4 cup honey

Nutrition Per Serving

Calories	412 cal
Protein	49 g
Sodium	119 mg

| Phosphorus | 357 mg |
| Potassium | 526 mg |

Directions

- Heat the oven to 350°F.
- Remove the turkey's giblets and neck.
- Fill the bird with celery, lemon, and onion.
- Use olive oil to rub the skin.
- Put the aluminum foil (2 sheets).
- With a separate sheet of foil, cover the top of the bird that you'll remove later.
- Wrap the foil's edges and place it on a rack; after that, roast it in the oven.
- While the turkey is cooking, melt the butter, thyme leaves, and chop sage finely.
- Add the butter with the bay leaves, chopped herbs, and honey.
- Simmer for 10 minutes, until the butter is lightly browned, and the bay leaves are removed.
- Raise the oven temperature to 500 degrees F when the turkey attains 145 to 155 degrees F, then remove the top foil and marinade turkey with the mixture of honey herb, every 5 to10 minutes or so.
- Using a thermometer, remove from the oven a shack with foil and leave to rest 30 minutes before carving when the turkey attains 160 degrees F.

79. Honey Molasses Pork

6 servings

Ingredients

- 2 tbsp. brown sugar
- 1/4 cup water
- 1/4 cup honey
- 1/4 cup balsamic vinegar
- 2 tbsp. Dijon mustard
- 2 tbsp. molasses
- 1 tbsp. canola oil
- 1 1/3 lbs. pork (3/4 inch thick)
- 1 tbsp. cornstarch
- 1/4 cup cold water

Nutrition Per Serving

| Calories | 241 cal |

Protein	21 g
Sodium	165 mg
Phosphorus	170 mg
Potassium	392 mg

Directions
- In a small bowl, add the brown sugar, water, honey, balsamic vinegar, Dijon mustard, and molasses and mix until well combined.
- Set it aside.
- Cut the pork into pieces that are 1/4 inch by 2 inches.
- Heat the oil over medium flame in a large frying pan.
- Add the pork and brown it from each side for 2 minutes.
- Add the honey molasses sauce, turn the heat down to medium-low, coat and cook for 15 minutes.
- In cold water, add the cornstarch and blend properly, then add it to the pork.
- Raise the heat to medium flame and bring to a boil, continuously stirring.
- Simmer for 5 minutes, uncovered, or till the sauce thickens.

80. Hungarian Goulash

6 servings
Ingredients
- 2 lbs. beef round steak
- 1/4 cup flour
- 1/4 cup oil or butter
- 1 1/2 cups chopped onions
- 1 cup beef stock, low sodium
- 2 tsp. sweet paprika
- 1 tbsp. wine vinegar or red wine

Nutrition Per Serving

Calories	450 cal
Protein	37 g
Sodium	200 mg
Phosphorus	300 mg
Dietary Fiber	30 g
Potassium	700 mg

Directions
- Cut the meat into cubes of 1 inch and cover with the flour.
- In a heavy pot, heat the oil or butter and then brown the meat on both sides.
- Mix in the onion and sauté.

- Add the stock. Add more if required. It should be dense and stew-like but easy to stir.
- Cover the pot.
- For 1 1/2 hours, simmer the meat.
- Take the meat out of the pot; keep it warm.
- To stock, add paprika and thicken it with corn starch or flour.
- Add vinegar or wine.
- Serve the goulash with noodles or spaetzle and salad.

81. Potato Soup, Irish Baked

6 servings

Ingredients
- 2 large potatoes
- 1/3 cup flour
- 4 cups skim milk
- 1/2 tsp. pepper
- 4 oz. cubed cheese
- 1/2 cup sour cream, fat-free

Nutrition Per Serving

Calories	275 cal
Protein	14 g
Sodium	226 mg
Phosphorus	261 mg
Dietary Fiber	7 g
Potassium	800 mg

Directions
- Bake the potatoes till tender at 400 degrees F or in a microwave till done.
- Let it cool down, then cut it lengthwise and scoop out the pulp.
- Brown flour on medium flame to a light brown color and progressively add the milk while stirring till it's blended.
- Add pepper and potato pulp.
- Cook it till bubbly and thick over medium heat, stirring frequently.
- Add the cheese and stir till the cheese melts.
- Remove from the flame and stir in the sour cream.

82. Italian Meatballs

12 (two meatballs each) servings

Ingredients
- 2 beaten large eggs
- 1.5 lbs. ground beef
- 1/2 tsp. black pepper
- 3 tbsp. parmesan cheese
- 1/2 cup oatmeal flakes, dry
- 1/2 tbsp. garlic powder
- 1/2 tbsp. olive oil
- 1/2 cup chopped onion
- 1 tsp. dried oregano

Nutrition Per Serving

Calories	163 cal
Protein	13 g
Sodium	72 mg
Phosphorus	125 mg
Potassium	199 mg

Directions
- Preheat the oven to 375°F.
- In a large bowl, combine all the ingredients and mix them.
- Place them on a baking sheet and roll into 1" balls.
- Bake for at least 10 - 15 minutes, till the meatballs are fully cooked.
- Set the meatballs in a crockpot or warming dish on a low flame setting to serve. Also, serve on the side with 2 tsp. of sauce.

83. Jammin' Jambalaya

6 servings

Ingredients
- 1/2 lb. shrimp, cooked, jumbo, tails removed
- 2 tsp. olive oil
- 1/2 large, chopped yellow onion
- 7 oz. sliced, smoked turkey sausage
- 3 cups chopped collard greens
- 1 large, chopped red bell pepper
- 1/4 tsp. cayenne pepper
- 2 minced garlic cloves
- 1 2/3 cups chicken broth
- 1/8 tsp. white pepper
- 1-2 tsp. Fresh thyme or 1/2 tsp. dry thyme

- 1/4 tsp. black pepper
- 2 bay leaves
- 1/2 tsp. oregano
- 1/2 cup rice (brown or white)
- 1/4 tsp. allspice

Nutrition Per Serving

Calories	200 cal
Protein	16 g
Sodium	400 mg
Phosphorus	170 mg
Dietary Fiber	6 g
Potassium	314 mg

Directions
- Heat the olive oil over a medium-high flame in a large skillet.
- Combine the turkey sausage, shrimp, bell pepper, onion, garlic, and collards.
- Cook, stirring occasionally, for 10 minutes.
- Get the remaining ingredients to a boil.
- Cover lower the flame to medium-low and cook till the rice is tender or for 20 minutes. (35 to 40 if brown rice is used).

Chapter 5: Dessert Recipes for Dialysis Diets

Are you having a desire for something sweet? If Yes, then you are in the right spot. You can always have dessert on a dialysis diet, and we have some tasty kidney-friendly recipes to consider. Note to review the recipes and nutritional info to align them with the meal planning strategies your dietician suggests. Believe it that you're going to discover a new favorite.

1. Pumpkin Strudel

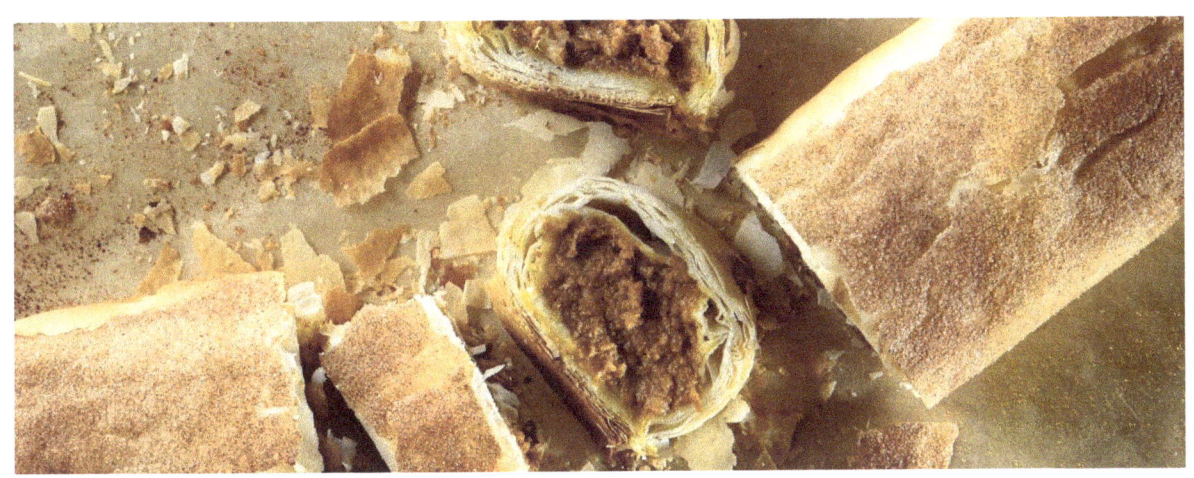

8 servings (1 serving = 1 slice)

Ingredients
- ⅛ tsp. grated nutmeg
- 12 sheets dough, phyllo (follow the package instructions for defrosting, if frozen)
- 1½ cups sodium-free, canned pumpkin, unsweetened
- 4 tbsp. sugar
- 1 tsp. Vanilla extract, pure
- ½ stick (4 tbsp.) butter, melted, unsalted
- ½ tsp. ground cinnamon

Nutrition Per Serving

Calories	180 cal
Protein	3 g
Sodium	141 mg
Phosphorus	39 mg
Dietary Fiber	2.0 g
Potassium	119 mg

Directions
- Preheat the oven to 375° F.

- Mix the nutmeg, canned pumpkin, vanilla extract, 2 tbsp. of sugar, and 1/2 tbsp. of cinnamon in a medium-sized bowl till well combined.
- Cover the bottom of the medium-sheet nonstick tray with melted butter by using a pastry brush. Layout a sheet of phyllo dough on a clean work surface and spray it with the butter. Brush other phyllo sheets with butter, then build a pile of buttered phyllo sheets. Hold the leftover phyllo dough sheets protected with plastic wrap till ready for usage, so they don't dry out. (Be mindful of saving some melted butter to spread on rolled filled strudel top, so go carefully while brushing in between the layers.)
- Spoon the mixture uniformly along with one of the stack's long edges once all the 12 sheets are used. Roll to the unfilled end from the filled end, ensuring that the seam-side heads down.
- Transfer the roll to the seam-side-down buttered sheet tray and rub with the remaining butter.
- Blend the remaining cinnamon and sugar in a small bowl. Spray it over the strudel's top and sides.
- Bake till golden brown or lightly toasted on the middle rack for about 12-15 minutes.
- Before slicing with a knife, take off the tray from the oven and make the toasted strudel to settle for 5 to 10 minutes, letting the center to sit. Serve.

2. Orange and Cinnamon Biscotti

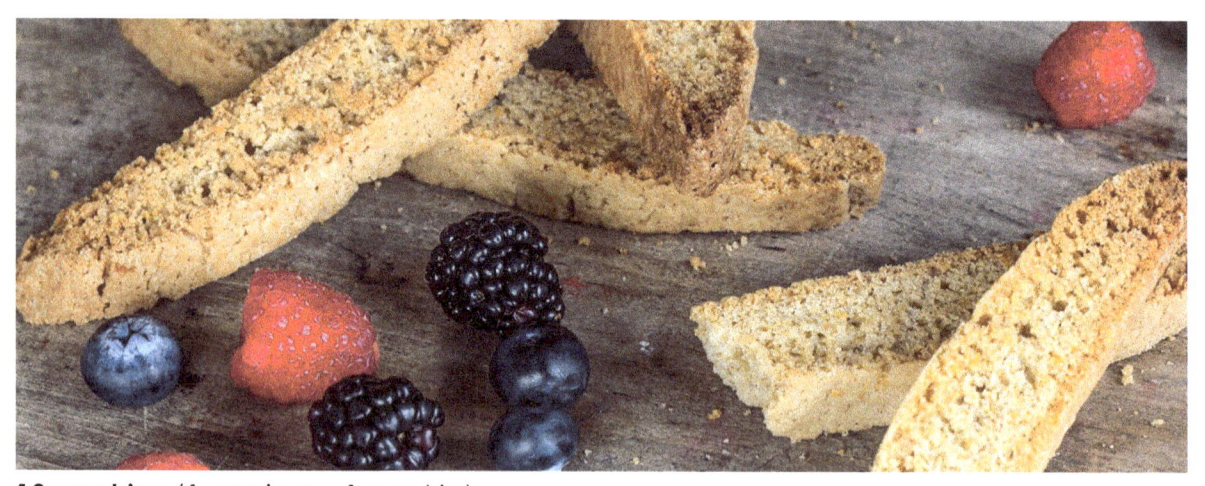

18 cookies (1 serving = 1 cookie)

Ingredients
- ½ cup butter, unsalted, room temperature
- 1 cup sugar
- 2 tsp. orange peel, grated
- 2 large eggs
- 2 cups flour, all-purpose
- 1 tsp. Vanilla extract

- ½ tsp. baking soda
- 1 tsp. Cream of tartar
- ¼ tsp. salt
- 1 tsp. ground cinnamon

Nutrition Per Serving

Calories	149 cal
Protein	2 g
Sodium	76 cal
Phosphorus	28 mg
Dietary Fiber	0.5 g
Potassium	53 mg

Directions

- Preheat the oven to 325° F.
- Spray with a nonstick cooking spray on 2 baking sheets.
- In a large bowl, beat the unsalted butter and sugar until well combined.
- Add the eggs, one at a time, bashing well after each one.
- Whisk in the vanilla and the orange peel.
- In a medium-size dish, combine the tartar cream, flour, baking soda, salt, and cinnamon.
- To the butter mixture, add the dry ingredients and combine until blended.
- Split the dough in two. Place each half on a sheet that has been prepared. Shape each half into a log form that is 3 inches wide and 3 quarters of an inch high with lightly floured hands. Bake for almost 35 minutes, till the dough logs, are smooth to the touch.
- Remove the oven's dough logs and cool for 10 minutes.
- Move logs to the surface of the work. Cut diagonally into 1/2-inch-thick slices utilizing serrated knives. On baking sheets, place cut side down.
- Bake for almost 12 minutes before the bottoms are golden.
- Turn over the biscotti; bake for almost 12 minutes more, till the bottoms are golden.
- Before serving, switch to a rack and let it cool.

3. Apple Cinnamon Filled Pastries

6 servings (1 serving = 1 pastry)

Ingredients

- Apple mixture:
- ¼ cup of light brown sugar
- 4 apples
- ¼ cup unsalted butter, melted (for buttering the phyllo pastry sheets)

- 2 tbsp. unsalted butter, firm
- ¼ tsp. nutmeg
- 1 tsp. cinnamon
- 1 package phyllo dough (6 sheets)
- ¼ tsp. cornstarch
- 2 tbsp. vanilla extract

Mix in a small bowl:
- 2 tbsp. cinnamon
- 3 tbsp. powdered sugar
- Optional: garnish with fresh mint sprigs, powdered sugar, and whipped cream

Nutrition Per Serving

Calories	280 cal
Protein	2 g
Sodium	97 mg
Phosphorus	33 mg
Dietary Fiber	5 g
Potassium	177 mg

Directions
Apple mixture:
- Preheat the oven to 350° F.
- Sauté the apples in the butter for 6 to 8 minutes in a wide sauté pan over medium-high flame.
- Stir in the cinnamon, brown sugar, and nutmeg. Cook for 3 or 4 more minutes.
- Mix the vanilla extract and cornstarch in a cup before it is dissolved. Stir in the apple mixture and simmer on a medium-high flame for an extra two minutes.
- Turn off the heat and set aside the mixture.

Phyllo dough pastries:
- Slightly grease a big 6-muffin tin pan.
- Dust each side with the melted butter and then sprinkle with the cinnamon mix and powdered sugar, beginning with the phyllo dough's first sheet. Proceed till all 6 sheets of cinnamon mix and sugar have been dusted and buttered, mounting one layer on top of the other as you go.
- Slice the stack into 6 squares each. Using a stack of squares to line the sides and bottom of each muffin cup, leaving several of the squares dangling over the muffin cup's edges.

- Fill with the apple mixture, each phyllo lined cup of muffin halfway to 3-quarters complete (this depends on how large the apples are sliced), ensuring that every phyllo lined cup of the muffin has similar quantities of apple mixture.
- In every muffin cup, fold the extra phyllo dough over apples.
- Bake for 8 to 10 minutes or till golden brown in the preheated oven at 350 ° F.
- Optional: Garnish with fresh sprigs of mint, powdered sugar, or whipped cream.

4. Very Berry Bread Pudding

10 servings (1 serving = 1 cup portion)

Ingredients
- 6 beaten eggs
- 8 cups challah bread, cubed
- 12-oz. bag of berry medley, frozen, thawed
- 2 cups of heavy cream
- Whipped cream
- 2 tsp. vanilla
- ½ cup sugar
- ½ tsp. cinnamon
- 1 tbsp. orange zest

Nutrition Per Serving

Calories	392 cal
Protein	9 g
Sodium	231 mg
Phosphorus	134 mg
Dietary Fiber	2.2 g
Potassium	172 mg

Directions
- Preheat the oven to 375° F.
- Whisk together the eggs, cream, sugar, orange zest, cinnamon, and vanilla till smooth.
- Mix the cubes of bread and the fruit with your hands.
- Pour into a greased/buttered pan, then bake for 35 minutes, covered with foil. Ensure it is unsalted before using butter.
- Take the foil off and bake for an extra 15 minutes.
- Turn the oven off and let it stay in the oven for 10 minutes.
- Cut, and serve with whipped cream on top.

5. Sunburst Lemon Bars

24 servings (1 serving = 1 bar)

Ingredients

Crust:
- 1 cup unsalted butter (2 sticks), room temperature
- ½ cup sugar, powdered
- 2 cups flour, all-purpose

Filling:
- 1½ cups sugar
- 4 eggs
- ½ tsp. cream of tartar
- ¼ cup flour, all-purpose
- ¼ cup lemon juice
- ¼ tsp. baking soda

Glaze:
- 2 tbsp. lemon juice
- 1 cup sifted powdered sugar

Nutrition Per Serving

Calories	200 cal
Protein	2 g
Sodium	27 mg
Phosphorus	32 mg
Dietary Fiber	0.3 g
Potassium	41 mg

Directions

Crust:
- Preheat the oven to 350° F.
- Combine the powdered sugar, flour, and 1 cup of butter in a big bowl. Mix together till crumbly. In a 9" x 13" baking pan, push the mixture onto the bottom.
- Bake for almost 15 to 20 minutes, till lightly browned.

Filling:
- Beat the eggs gently in a medium-sized bowl.
- Combine the flour, tartar cream, sugar, and baking soda in another bowl. In the eggs, add the dry mixture. Then to the egg mixture, add the lemon juice and mix till thickened slightly.
- Pour it over the crust and bake for an additional 20 minutes or till the filling is set.
- Take it out of the oven and cool.

Glaze:
- Mix the lemon juice steadily into the powdered sugar in a small bowl till it is spreadable. As desired, add less or more lemon juice.
- Spread over the filling that has been cooled. Let the glaze settle and cut into 24 bars afterward. Hold the leftover lemon bars in the freezer.

6. Ginger- Lemon-Coconut Cookies

2 dozen (1 serving = 1 cookie) cookies

Ingredients
- ½ cup sugar
- ½ cup butter (1 stick), unsalted
- ½ tsp. baking soda
- 1 egg
- 1 tbsp. lemon zest
- 1 cup unsweetened, toasted coconut
- 2 tbsp. lemon juice
- 1 ¼ cups flour
- 1 tbsp. chopped and peeled or grated, fresh ginger

Nutrition Per Serving

Calories	97 cal
Protein	1 g
Sodium	40 mg
Phosphorus	17 mg
Dietary Fiber	0.4 g
Potassium	27 mg

Directions
- Preheat the oven to 350° F.
- Spread the unsweetened coconut on the baking sheet tray and bake for almost 5 to10 minutes till the edges are light brown.
- Take it out of the oven and put it aside in a bowl.
- Cream the sugar and butter until fluffy and light using an electric mixer. Add the egg, lemon juice, lemon zest and chopped ginger and blend until smooth.
- Sift the flour and the baking soda together. In the butter mixture, stir the flour mixture and combine until fully mixed.
- For at least 30 minutes, cover and wait.
- Scoop out balls that are tablespoon-size and coil them in toasted coconut. Use a slightly lubricated baking sheet tray to put balls almost 2 inches apart.

- Bake for 10 to 12 minutes till the edges are slightly brown. Remove and cool on a cool surface or counter.

7. Cranberry Fruit Bars, Dried

24 bars (1 serving = 1 bar)

Ingredients
Topping:
- 1 tsp. baking powder
- ½ cup flour, all-purpose
- ¾ cup of sugar
- 1 cup cranberries, dried
- 1 tsp. vanilla extract
- 4 eggs, large
- Optional: Powdered sugar (for dusting)

Crust:
- 1 1/3 cups of sugar
- 1 ½ cups flour, all-purpose
- ¾ cup butter (1 1/2 sticks), unsalted

Nutrition Per Serving

Calories	190 cal
Protein	2 g
Sodium	34 mg
Phosphorus	34 mg
Dietary Fiber	0.6 g
Potassium	28 mg

Directions
- Preheat the oven to 350° F.
- Stir together the flour and sugar in a medium-sized bowl; slice in unsalted butter till the mixture holds together. Pat into the 9" x 13" ungreased baking pan. Bake till slightly browned, for 10 minutes.
- In a small bowl, sift the baking powder and flour together to prepare the topping. Put the dried cranberries in. Set aside.
- Mix the sugar, vanilla, and eggs in a medium-size bowl. Add a mixture of flour. Add onto baked crust. For 20 to 25 minutes, bake.
- While warm, cut into 24 bars and brush with powdered sugar.

8. Molten Chocolate Mint Brownies

12 brownies (1 serving = 2.5oz.)

Ingredients
- 1 box of Betty Crocker brownie mix, not supreme
- 12 Andes chocolates, mint
- Optional garnish: cocoa powder (sweetened or unsweetened), powdered sugar, fresh mint sprigs

Nutrition Per Serving

Calories	307 cal
Protein	3 g
Sodium	147 mg
Phosphorus	61 mg
Dietary Fiber	0 g
Potassium	120 mg

Directions
- Preheat the oven and ready the mixture of brownie according to the box's instructions.
- Prepare a lining or finely greased 12 cup muffin tin and flour the sides and bottom. Pour the brownie mixture onto the pan and bake for 25 minutes. Take the brownies out of the oven and place one bit of mint candy in the middle and bake for an extra 5 minutes. Turn the oven off and take it. For 5–10 minutes, let cool.
- Take the brownie cupcakes out of the pan, then serve.
- Optional: Dust with powdered sugar and cocoa powder and garnish with the fresh mint

9. Cream Cheese Sugar Cookies

48 servings (1 serving = 1 cookie)

Ingredients
- 1 cup softened, unsalted butter
- 1 cup of sugar
- 1 egg, large, separated
- 3 oz. softened cream cheese
- ¼ tsp. almond extract
- ½ tsp. salt
- 2¼ cups flour, all-purpose
- ½ tsp. vanilla extract
- Optional: garnish with colored sugar

Nutrition Per Serving

Calories	79 cal
Protein	1 g
Sodium	33 mg
Phosphorus	11 mg
Dietary Fiber	0 g
Potassium	11 mg

Directions

- Place the butter, sugar, cream cheese, almond extract, salt, egg yolk, and vanilla extract in a large bowl. Blend thoroughly. Stir in the flour till it is well-mixed.
- Chill the cookie dough in the fridge for 2 hours.
- Preheat the oven to 350° F.
- Roll out the pastry, one third at a time to 1/4-inch width, on a thinly floured board. Break using thinly floured cookie cutters into ideal forms.
- Place them on ungreased cookie sheets 1 inch apart. Dust with egg white, which is slightly beaten and sprinkle with the colored sugar or leave the cookies plain if desired.
- For 7 to 9 minutes or till light golden brown, bake the cream cheese cookies. Before serving, let it cool completely.

10. Ice Cream Pumpkin Pie

8 servings

Ingredients

- 1 cup pumpkin, canned
- 1 pint or 2 cups softened vanilla ice cream.
- 1/2 tsp. ginger
- 3/4 cup of sugar
- 1/4 tsp. nutmeg
- 1/2 tsp. cinnamon
- 1 9" baked pie shell
- 1 cup whipped topping

Nutrition Per Serving

Calories	275 cal
Protein	3 g
Sodium	118 mg
Phosphorus	51 mg
Potassium	90 mg

Directions
- Mix all the ingredients in the food processor, except the pie shell, till well mixed.
- Pour the mixture into the baked pie shell and freeze till firm.

11. Sweet Cherry Cobbler

12 servings

Ingredients

Cherry Filling
- 2/3 cup sugar, granulated
- 5 cups halved and pitted red cherries, sweet, about 1.7 lbs.
- 1/4 tsp. salt
- 1/4 tsp. almond extract
- 2 tbsp. cornstarch
- 1 tsp. vanilla extract
- 2 tbsp. lemon juice

Cobbler Topping
- 1/2 cup sugar
- 1 cup flour, all-purpose
- 1/2 cup cold milk, non-fat
- 1/4 tsp. salt
- 1 tsp. baking powder
- 2 tbsp. unsalted, cubed, and cold butter
- 1/4 tsp. ground cinnamon

Nutrition Per Serving

Calories	117 cal
Protein	2 g
Sodium	103 mg
Phosphorus	65 mg
Dietary Fiber	2 g
Potassium	186 mg

Directions
Preheat your oven to 450°F.

Cherry Filling
- Prepare the cherries. To pit the cherries, you may split the cherries in two, either remove the pits or use a solid straw-like one with a reusable plastic cup. Force the straw up from the bottom of the cherry through the tip. The pit's going to pop straight out. Cut the cherries from the middle, then. This procedure is a little sloppy but preparing the cherries in half can reduce the time.

- In a big saucepan, put the sugar, cherries, salt, cornstarch, and whisk in the lemon juice, almond extract and vanilla extract.
- Carry to a boil on medium flame and cook for around 5 to 7 minutes till the cherries are tenderized and the juices are thickened.
- Pour the filling of the cherry into an ungreased baking pan of 8-inches. (Round or square.)

Cobbler Topping
- In a medium bowl, put the sugar, flour, baking powder, cinnamon, and salt and stir until combined.
- Slice in the butter using a pastry blender or fork, so the mixture looks like coarse crumbs.
- In limited quantities, add the milk slowly, only enough to lubricate the dough. (Maybe you might not need all the milk.)
- Drop the spoonful of dough on the top of the filling a cookie dough scoop or a soup spoon. Leave several airflow gaps such that between the scoops of the dough, the filling will bubble up.
- Bake till the top is golden brown, for 10 to 15 minutes. Using a toothpick, test for doneness. Upon thoroughly cooking the dough topping, the toothpick must be clean.
- Serve warm, or up to 1 week you can keep in the fridge. To Reheat, let it stand for at least 30 minutes to one hour at room temperature and reheat for 10 to 15 minutes at 350 °F.

12. Mini pineapple cake

12 servings
Ingredients
- 1/3 cup brown sugar, packed
- 3 tbsp. melted butter, unsalted
- 6 cherries, sliced into halves, fresh and pitted
- 12 canned pineapple slices, unsweetened
- 2/3 cup milk, fat-free
- 1/4 tsp. salt
- 2/3 cup sugar
- 1 egg
- 3 tbsp. canola oil
- 1/2 tsp. vanilla extract
- 1 tsp. lemon juice
- 1-1/4 tsp. baking powder
- 1-1/3 cups of cake flour

Nutrition Per Serving

Calories	193 cal
Protein	3 g
Sodium	131 mg
Phosphorus	88 mg
Dietary Fiber	1 g
Potassium	169 mg

Directions
- Pour batter into a muffin pan with 12 servings. Square pan for baking.
- Sprinkle each segment with a little bit of brown sugar.
- Press one slice of pineapple into each segment to create a cup shape. In the middle of each pineapple slice, put one half of the cherry (cut side must be facing up) and set aside.
- Beat the oil, milk, sugar, egg and extracts in a wide bowl until well mixed. Combine the baking powder, salt, and flour; beat into the sugar mixture till mixed. In a muffin pan, mix into the prepared batter.
- For 35 to 40 minutes, bake at 350°F or till a toothpick comes out clean. Invert the muffin pan directly and transfer the cooked cakes into a serving tray. If required, you may use a butter knife or a tiny spatula around the edges to gently extract them from the pan. Serve it warm.

13. Dutch Apple Pancake

4 servings

Ingredients
- 3 large, sliced, and peeled Granny Smith apples
- 2 tbsp. unsalted butter
- 1 tsp. ground cinnamon
- 6 tbsp. granulated sugar
- 1/2 cup flour, all-purpose
- 3 eggs
- 1 tbsp. sour cream
- 1/2 cup milk
- 1 tsp. lemon zest, grated
- 1/4 tsp. salt

Nutrition Per Serving

Calories	339 kcals
Protein	8 g
Sodium	217 mg

Phosphorus	139 mg
Dietary Fiber	5 g
Potassium	290 mg

Directions

- Melt the butter in an ovenproof pan over medium-high flame.
- Add the cinnamon, sugar, and apples; sauté and mix for 3 to 5 minutes. Remove from the flame.
- Beat the eggs in a bowl until frothy. Add the milk, flour, sour cream, zest, and salt.
- Beat until it forms a smooth batter.
- Pour the apples over and bake till golden brown and puffed in a 400 degrees F oven for about 25 minutes.
- Slice into a wedge, then serve directly from the pan.
- Optional: Brush with powdered sugar or drizzle with the honey.

14. Butterscotch Apple Crisp

9 servings

Ingredients

- 1 tbsp. lemon juice
- 6 cups sliced and peeled cooking apples
- 2 tsp. ground cinnamon
- 1/2 cup unsalted butter or margarine
- 1 tbsp. water
- 1/2 cup flour, all-purpose
- 1/4 cup of light brown sugar
- 1 (3-1/4 oz.) butterscotch pudding, package, and pie filling mix (but not instant)
- 1/2 cup rolled oats

Nutrition Per Serving

Calories	234 kcals
Protein	2 g
Sodium	53 mg
Phosphorus	39 mg
Dietary Fiber	3 g
Potassium	143 mg

Directions

- Heat the oven to 375 F. Place the apples in a square 8 or 9-inch pan. Spray with the lemon juice, 1 tsp. of cinnamon, and water.
- In a small bowl, add the brown sugar, rolled oats, flour, the pudding, and the remaining cinnamon, then mix.

- Melt the butter or margarine. Mix till crumbly with the pudding mixture. Sprinkle over the apples. Bake till the apples are tender or bake for 40 to 45 minutes. Serve cooled or warm
- Serve with the non-dairy dessert or non-dairy creamer, if needed.

15. Low Sodium Pound Cake

Serving Size: 1/9 cake
Ingredients
- 3/4 cup Sugar
- 1/4 lb. unsalted Butter
- 1 1/4 cup bread flour
- 2 large, slightly beaten eggs
- 3 oz. Milk

Nutrition Per Serving

Calories	243 cal
Protein	3.7 g
Sodium	18 mg
Phosphorus	45 mg
Dietary Fiber	0.6 g
Potassium	47 mg

Directions
- Cream the butter and add the sugar gradually.
- Strike till fluffy.
- Add the flour, eggs, and milk.
- Mix thoroughly.
- Line 18×13 in the pan with the pan paper.
- Bake for 30 minutes at 375 F.

16. Apple Cake with Sauce, Cinnamon Yogurt

12 servings (serving size:1 slice)
Ingredients
- 2 cups golden, chopped, unpeeled delicious apples
- 3/4 cups of apples and sugar
- 3/4 cup flour
- 1 cup packed light brown sugar
- 1 tsp. baking soda
- 3/4 cup flour, whole wheat

- ½ tsp. salt
- 1 tsp. vanilla
- 1 tsp. cinnamon
- 1/4 tsp. ground cloves
- 1/4 tsp. ginger
- 1/4 cup vegetable oil
- 2 large, lightly beaten eggs

Nutrition Per Serving

Calories	186 kcals
Protein	4 g
Sodium	156 mg
Phosphorus	86 mg
Potassium	172 mg

Directions
- Combine 3/4 of the sugar and apples; leave and let it stand for at least 45 minutes.
- Combine the flour, baking soda, whole wheat flour, 1 tsp. of cinnamon, salt, ginger, and ground cloves.
- In the apple mixture, whisk in 2 big eggs, vanilla, and vegetable oil.
- Add the mixture of flour and the remaining apples; thoroughly mix.
- Pour into a lightly floured lubricated pan; bake at 350F for at least 40 to 45 minutes.
- Let it cool for 10 minutes on a wire rack; unmold.
- Spray 1 tbsp. Confectioners' sugar over the cake.
- Combine one cup of low-fat plain yogurt and 1 1/2 tsp of cinnamon.
- Serve the mixture of yogurt with the cake.

17. Carmel-Filled Butterscotch Cookies

12 cookies

Ingredients
- 1 cup sugar, light brown
- ½ cup unsalted margarine, (1 stick)
- 3 tbsp. of egg alternative (or one large egg)
- ½ tsp. baking soda
- 3 tbsp. granulated sugar
- 1-3/4 cups flour, all-purpose
- 2 tsp. vanilla extract
- ½ tsp. baking powder
- ½ bag of caramel cubes

- 1-1/2 cups of butterscotch morsels

Nutrition Per Serving

Calories	210 kcals
Protein	1.5 g
Sodium	67 mg
Phosphorus	35 mg
Dietary Fiber	0.3 g
Potassium	82 mg

Directions
- Preheat the oven to 350°F.
- Use an electric mixer to cream the butter with sugars at medium speed till fluffy (almost 30 seconds).
- Beat in the vanilla extract and the egg for a further 30 seconds.
- Sift the dried ingredients together in a mixing bowl and mix in the butter mixture for almost 15 seconds at low speed. Stir the chips of butterscotch in.
- Drop the cookie dough on a cookie sheet coated with parchment paper or a buttered cookie sheet, approximately 3 inches apart with one tbsp. Ice cream scoop. Put one caramel square in the middle and top with another tbsp. of dough.
- Roll these in your hand to make them a smooth, even ball.
- Bake till well browned around the edges for almost 12 to 20 minutes. Like most kinds of cookies, these cookies will stay somewhat thick and won't spread out.
- NOTE: On the cookie sheet, let the cookies cool absolutely. Much of the caramel might have fallen to the bottom, so this is an important move to prevent breaking the cookies.
- Microwave 1 or 2 at a time for 10 seconds to thoroughly enjoy the cookies for the next few days.

18. Spicy Angel Cake

18 slices (serving size: 1–inch slice)

Ingredients
- 1 tsp. cinnamon, ground
- 1 package Angel food cake mix
- 1/4 tsp. cloves, ground
- 1/4 tsp. ginger, ground
- 1/2 tsp. nutmeg, ground

Nutrition Per Serving

Calories	112 cal
Protein	2.5 g

Sodium	55 mg
Phosphorus	36 mg
Dietary Fiber	0 g
Potassium	34 mg

Directions
- Sift all the ingredients together.
- Prepare and bake according to box instructions.
- Invert.
- Cool in the pan thoroughly
- Remove.
- Slice into pieces of 1 inch.
- Serve with fresh pineapple and strawberries and a whipped topping.

19. Easy Fruit Dip

8 servings

Ingredients
- 1 jar or 7 oz. marshmallow cream
- 1 package or 8 oz. cream cheese
- 1 tbsp. orange peel, dried

Nutrition Per Serving

Calories	183 cal
Protein	2 g
Sodium	104 mg
Phosphorus	31 mg
Dietary Fiber	0 g
Potassium	36 mg

Directions
- Mix all the ingredients till the mixture is smooth.
- Serve with fresh fruits such as grapes, strawberries, and apples.

20. Crispy Butterscotch Cookies

12 cookies

Ingredients
- 1/2 cup brown sugar, packed
- 1/2 cup margarine
- 3 tbsp. egg alternative (or one egg)
- 1/2 cup sugar

- 1 cup butterscotch chips
- 1 tsp. vanilla extract
- 1 tbsp. milk
- 1 tsp. baking powder
- 1 cup + 3 tbsp. flour, all-purpose
- 1 cup wheat cream
- 1.2 tsp. ground cinnamon

Nutrition Per Serving

Calories	100 cal
Protein	0.7 g
Sodium	46 mg
Phosphorus	22 mg
Potassium	32 mg

Directions

- Preheat the oven to 350 degrees F.
- Grease the cookie sheet.
- Whisk together the sugar and butter till creamy.
- Beat till fluffy and add the milk, vanilla, and egg.
- Toss the baking powder, cinnamon, and flour together.
- Add to the butter mixture: blend well.
- Stir in the butterscotch chips and cereal.
- Drop by level tbsp. onto the prepared cookie sheet.
- Bake for 9 to 12 minutes, or till browned lightly.
- Let it stand for a minute on the cookie sheet before placing it onto the racks to cool.
- Serve.

21. Chocolate Covered Strawberries

18 portions (serving size: 2 each)

Ingredients

- 1 tbsp. Corn syrup
- 1/2 cup Chocolate chips, Semi-sweet
- 1 qt. washed and dried Strawberries
- 5 tbsp. Margarine

Nutrition Per Serving

Calories	69 cal
Protein	0.5 g
Sodium	40 mg

Phosphorus	14 mg
Dietary Fiber	0.7 g
Potassium	70 mg

Directions

- Over the low flame, melt the chocolate chips, corn syrup, and margarine.
- Until smooth, stir.
- Remove from the flame; put in the pan of water.
- Dip in strawberries into the chocolate; put on a waxed paper.
- Refrigerate.

22. Pineapple Cream Cake

18 servings

Ingredients

- 1/4 cup sugar
- 1 8-oz. softened cream cheese
- 1 8-oz. drained and canned, crushed pineapple
- 5 eggs, large
- 1/3 cup vegetable oil
- 1 box of yellow cake mix (about 18 oz.)
- 1 tsp. vanilla flavoring
- 1 cup water

Nutrition Per Serving

Calories	233 kcals
Protein	4 g
Sodium	250 mg
Phosphorus	41 mg
Dietary Fiber	0 g
Potassium	48 mg

Directions

- Preheat the oven to the recommended temperature on the cake mix box.
- Combine the cream cheese, two eggs, and sugar in a small bowl, stirring well. Stir in and put aside the drained pineapple.
- Combine the water, yellow cake mix, vanilla flavoring, the remaining 3 eggs, and oil in a large bowl. Beat at high speed for two minutes using an electric mixer.
- Spray with cooking spray, a 9 X 3.5-inch tube pan, then cover it with flour.
- Add the cream cheese mixture to the cake batter and mix well. Then mix the batter into the floured and greased pan.

- Bake just until the middle is ready for 55 to 65 minutes. The doneness measure is achieved by sticking a butter knife into the middle of the cake. For 10 minutes, cool in the pan.

23. Sugarless Pecan and Raisin Cookies

42 cookies

Ingredients
- 2 tsp. of baking powder
- 1 3/4 cup flour
- 1/2 tsp. Cinnamon
- 1/2 tsp. Salt
- 1/2 tsp. grated orange rind
- 3/4 cup canned, unsweetened orange juice
- 1 egg
- 1/4 cup oil
- 1/2 cup raisins
- 1/2 cup pecans

Nutrition Per Serving

Calories	6 cal
Protein	0.8 g
Sodium	44 mg
Phosphorus	15 mg
Dietary Fiber	0.3 g
Potassium	34 mg

Directions
- Combine the baking powder, salt, flour, and cinnamon.
- Add the remaining ingredients.
- Mix thoroughly.
- On an un-greased baking sheet, drop by tsp.
- Bake at 375 F for at least 15 to 20 minutes.

24. Sugar Cookies

40 medium-sized cookies

Ingredients
- 1-1/2 tsp. baking powder
- 2 cups of sifted flour
- 1/2 cup margarine, unsalted

- 1/2 tsp. salt
- 1 well-beaten egg
- 1 cup sugar
- 1 tbsp. non-dairy creamer
- 1 tsp. vanilla

Nutrition Per Serving

Calories	631 kcals
Protein	1 g
Sodium	21 mg
Phosphorus	11 mg
Dietary Fiber	0 g
Potassium	9 mg

Directions

- Sift 1-1/2 cups of baking powder, salt, and flour together.
- Cream the margarine; gradually add the sugar and cream till fluffy and light. Add the non-dairy creamer, egg, red food coloring, and egg. Add the sifted dry ingredients. Then steadily add the rest of the 1/2 cup of flour till the dough is stiff enough to cope. Chill for 1 hour at least.
- Roll on lightly floured board 1/8 inch thick, shape (with hand or by cookie cutter) and put it on floured sheets of cookie. Add sugar to sprinkle. Bake in the oven at 375 F for 8 to10 minutes.

25. Strawberry Pie

8 servings

Ingredients

- 4 cups strawberries
- 2 tbsp. lemon juice
- 1 single crust, 9-inch, unbaked pie shell
- 3 tbsp. cornstarch
- 1 cup sugar

Nutrition Per Serving

Calories	246 kcals
Protein	2 g
Sodium	118 mg
Phosphorus	30 mg
Dietary Fiber	3 g
Potassium	146 mg

Directions

Bake the pie shell till it's brown; then cool
- Mash two cups of strawberries and mix them with milk, lemon juice and cornstarch. In a saucepan, over medium flame, prepare the mixture. Constantly stir till it is clear and thick. Cool
- Cut and add the leftover strawberries to the cooled mixture. Pour it into the pie shell.
- Wrap with the plastic sheet and place in the refrigerator till completely cooled.
- Serve, if wanted, with whipped topping.

26. Spicy Raisin Cookies

45 Cookies

Ingredients
- 1/2 cup white sugar
- 1/2 cup butter or margarine, unsalted (at room temperature)
- 1 large, beaten egg
- 1/2 cup firmly packed, light brown sugar
- 1/4 tsp. almond extract
- 1/2 tsp. vanilla extract
- 1/2 tsp. baking soda
- 1-1/2 cups flour, all-purpose
- 1/2 tsp. ground nutmeg
- 1/2 tsp. ground cinnamon
- 1/2 cup raisins
- 1/8 tsp. ground cloves
- 1/4 tsp. ground ginger
- 1 cup well-drained fruit cocktail in syrup
- 1/8 tsp. salt

Nutrition Per Serving

Calories	61 kcals
Protein	1 g
Sodium	17 mg
Phosphorus	8 mg
Dietary Fiber	0 g
Potassium	34 mg

Directions
- Preheat the oven to 375 F. Slightly flour and grease the baking sheets.

- Cream the margarine in a big bowl with white sugar. Blend them in brown sugar. Add the almond extracts, vanilla and egg; beat till smooth.
- Combine the dry ingredients and add them to the creamy mixture. Stir in the raisins and fruit cocktail.
- Drop by heaping tsp. onto the baking sheets. Bake for almost 11 to 12 minutes, till lightly golden. Cool for 2 to 3 minutes on baking sheets. To cool, transfer to the wire racks.
- Store it in an airtight container.

27. Almond Pecan Caramel Corn

10 servings

Ingredients

- 2 cups almonds, unblanched
- 3/4 cup of popcorn kernels or 20 cups of popped Popcorn
- 1 cup sugar, granulated
- 1 cup pecan halves
- 1/2 cup of corn syrup
- 1 cup butter, unsalted
- 1 tsp. baking soda
- Pinch of tartar cream

Nutrition Per Serving

Calories	604 cal
Protein	8 g
Sodium	149 mg
Phosphorus	201 mg
Dietary Fiber	4 g
Potassium	285 mg

Directions

- Layer the cooked Popcorn uniformly with pecans and almonds in a large roasting pan.
- Stir together the butter, sugar, corn syrup, and tartar cream in a big, heavy saucepan.
- Bring to a boil on a medium-high flame, continuously stirring. Let it simmer without stirring for 5 minutes.
- Take it off the heat and stir in the baking soda.
- Pour the caramel uniformly over the mixture of Popcorn, stirring until well coated.
- Bake for 1 hour at 200 degrees F stirring after every 10 minutes.
- Let it cool, sometimes stirring. Store for up to one week in an airtight container.

28. Apple with Cream Cheese Torte

10 servings

Ingredients

- 3/4 cup sugar (divided into 1/4 cups)
- 1/2 cup softened unsalted butter
- 8 oz. softened cream cheese
- 1 cup flour
- 1 tsp. vanilla
- 1 egg
- 1/2 tsp. cinnamon
- 3-4 medium, thinly sliced apples

Nutrition Per Serving

Calories	298 cal
Protein	4 g
Sodium	176 mg
Phosphorus	34 mg
Potassium	102 mg

Directions

- Preheat the oven to 450°F.
- Cream 1/4 cup of sugar and butter in a medium-sized bowl.
- Blend it with flour.
- Press it into a springform pan.
- Whisk together the 1/4 cup of the sugar, cream cheese, vanilla, and egg till smooth.
- Spread it into the pan.
- Toss the remaining cinnamon and 1/4 cup of sugar with the apples.
- Arrange apples over the filling of cheese.
- For 10 minutes, bake.
- Reduce the oven temperature to 400 °F and bake for a further 25 to 30 minutes till the apples are softened, and the filling is firm.

29. Asian Pear Crisp

6-8 servings

Ingredients

- 1/2 cup all-purpose flour, unbleached
- 3/4 cup chopped nuts
- 4 tbsp. divided, granulated sugar
- 1/4 cup sugar, light brown

- 1/8 tsp. ground nutmeg
- 1/4 tsp. ground cinnamon
- 1 tbsp. cornstarch
- 5 tbsp. unsalted butter
- 3 lbs. peeled and cored Asian pears
- Juice from one lemon

Nutrition Per Serving

Calories	401 cal
Protein	6 g
Sodium	53 mg
Phosphorus	86 mg
Potassium	127 mg

Directions
- Preheat the oven to 375°F.
- In a food processor, combine the nuts, brown sugar, flour, 2 tsp. of granulated sugar, nutmeg, and cinnamon.
- Pour the melted butter over the mixture and blend till the mixture looks like wet sand.
- In a large bowl, mix the remaining 2 tsp. of granulated sugar, lemon juice, and cornstarch.
- Peel the pears. Slice into wedges and split in half.
- Toss the sugar mixture with the pears and move to an 8-inch baking dish (square).
- Sprinkle the toppings with pears.
- Bake for almost 45 minutes, till the fruit bubbles around the edges and the top is deep golden brown.
- Cool for about 15 minutes on a wire rack. Serve.

30. Asian Pear Tort

8-10 servings

Ingredients
- 1 1/2 cups almonds and 1/4 cup for garnish
- 2/3 cup sugar
- 1 1/2 cups flour
- 1 tsp. cinnamon
- 1 tbsp. lemon zest
- 1/2 cup apple, lemon marmalade

- 1 cup, unsalted, cold butter, sliced into cubes
- 1 tsp. almond extract
- 2-3 Asian pears
- 2 egg yolks
- powdered sugar and marishino cherry for garnish

Nutrition Per Serving

Calories	426 cal
Protein	8 g
Sodium	9 mg
Phosphorus	158 mg
Dietary Fiber	31 g
Potassium	246 mg

Directions
- Preheat the oven to 350°.
- Pulse 1 1/2 cups of nuts, sugar, flour, cinnamon, and lemon in a food processor till the nuts are perfectly chopped.
- Add butter, almond extract, and egg yolks.
- Pulse to blend.
- Grease the sides and bottom of the 9" spring shape pan, load with the dough, and press up to the sides. Set aside 1/4-1/2 cups of batter.
- Slice about 1/4" thick Asian Pears.
- Starting at the middle of the batter, from the center, layer slices in a consecutive ring. Make two complete rings around the top of the torte.
- To create a crust of sorts, scatter the reserved batter over the side of the torte and the end of pears.
- Melt the jelly in the microwave for 1 minute and brush it over the Asian pear slices.
- Sprinkle the remaining sliced almonds on the center and edges.
- Bake for 30 to 35 minutes or so.
- Before opening the Spring Form Pan, let it cool.
- Sprinkle with the powdered sugar and garnish with the maraschino cherry in the middle.

31. Blueberry Squares

16 servings
Ingredients
- 1 cup oats
- 1 1/2 cups of flour
- 1 cup sugar

- 1 tsp. cinnamon
- 3 cups blueberries
- 1 1/2 sticks or 3/4 cup butter, melted (unsalted if possible)
- 3 tbsp. cornstarch
- zest of 1 lemon
- 1 cup water
- 3/4 cup of sugar

Nutrition Per Serving

Calories	247 cal
Protein	2 g
Sodium	3 mg
Phosphorus	17 mg
Potassium	38 mg

Directions
- Preheat the oven to 350°F.
- Combine the oats, flour, sugar, cinnamon, and butter in a medium bowl, till crumbly.
- In a square pan of 9 inches, press half of the oat mixture and flour.
- With the lemon zest, toss the blueberries and coat the bottom of the pan.
- In a safe microwave bowl, mix the sugar and cornstarch, whisk in water steadily and heat till just boiling.
- Pour the mixture of cornstarch/water/sugar over the blueberries.
- Over the top, pour the remaining oat/flour mixture.
- Cook for 45 minutes to 1 hour.

32. Blueberry Whipped Pie

9 servings

Ingredients
- 1 tsp. cinnamon
- 2 cups of graham cracker crumbs
- 8 oz. softened cream cheese
- 1/2 cup melted butter, unsalted.
- 1 tsp. vanilla extract
- 1/4 cup sugar, granulated.
- 3 cups blueberries
- 8 oz. whipped cream, non-dairy

- 2 tsp. lemon juice

Nutrition Per Serving

Calories	343 cal
Protein	4 g
Sodium	197 mg
Phosphorus	38 mg
Potassium	59 mg

Directions
- Preheat the oven to 375°F.
- Combine the cinnamon, melted butter, and the graham cracker crumbs in a medium bowl.
- To form a crust, push the mixture uniformly into the bottom of the square or round baking dish of 9 inches.
- Bake the crust for at least 7 minutes and let it cool.
- Use the electric mixer in a large bowl to blend the cream cheese and sugar till smooth.
- Mix the lemon juice and vanilla extract.
- Fold in whipped topping gently; after that, fold in blueberries.
- Spread the mixture equally over the crust.
- Cover and cool for at least 1 hour in the refrigerator.

33. Caramel Apple Pound Cake

12 servings

Ingredients
- 1 box sugar-free cake mix, or yellow cake mix.
- 3 medium, peeled, Granny Smith apples, diced and cored.
- 12 egg whites
- 1/4 cup sugar-free or regular caramel flavored syrup
- 3/4 cup of flour
- 2 tbsp. water
- 1/4 cup vegetable oil

Nutrition Per Serving

Calories	300 cal
Protein	7 g
Sodium	319 mg
Phosphorus	160 mg
Potassium	141 mg

Directions

- Preheat the oven to 350°F. For 6 minutes on a high or till they are tender, microwave the diced apples. Mash till applesauce and let it cool down to room temperature.
- Add the cake mix, egg whites, flour, vegetable oil, apple mixture, caramel flavoring, and water into a mixing bowl. Mix for a minute at low speed, scraping the bowl's sides. Then blend at medium speed for 2 minutes.
- Onto 2 greased loaf pans or a baking dish of 9 by 13 inches, pour the batter. For 30 to 45 minutes, bake. When a toothpick that is stuck in the center comes out clean, the cake is done. Before serving, dust it with powdered sugar after the cake is cooled.

34. Caramel Custard

6 servings

Ingredients
- 2 tbsp. water
- 2 tbsp. sugar
- 4 drops of vanilla extract
- 6 eggs
- 3 cups 2% milk
- 1/2 cup plus 2 tbsp. sugar

Nutrition Per Serving

Calories	215 cal
Protein	9 g
Sodium	116 mg
Phosphorus	194 mg
Dietary Fiber	6 g
Potassium	241 mg

Directions
- Place the water and sugar in a heat-proof dish and put in a microwave to prepare the caramel.
- Cook on high for 4 minutes or till the sugar is caramelized.
- Melt the water and sugar in the pan till pale gold in color, to make it on the stove.
- Pour in a baking dish or a 5 cups shouffle.
- Let it cool.
- Preheat the oven to 350°F.
- Break the eggs into a medium mixing bowl to prepare the custard; whisk till frothy.
- Add in vanilla extract.
- Add the sugar gradually and then milk by continuously whisking.
- Over the top of the caramel, pour the custard.
- Cook for 35 to 40 minutes in a preheated oven.

- Remove from the oven and cool for approximately 30 minutes, or till set.
- Loosen the custard with a knife from the side of the dish. On top of the souffle dish, put the serving dish upside down and invert, providing a slight shake.
- Arrange the choice of fruit around the caramel. Options like banana slices and orange ring, or consider blueberries, raspberries, or strawberries for a lesser potassium option.

35. Carrot Muffins

12 servings

Ingredients
- 1/2 cup of whole wheat flour
- 1/2 cup flour, all-purpose
- 1/4 cup seed, ground flax (optional)
- 1/2 cup oats
- 3/4 tsp. baking soda
- 3/4 tsp. baking powder
- 1/2 tsp. ginger (optional)
- 3/4 tsp. cinnamon
- 1/2 cup vegetable oil
- 1/2 cup of brown sugar
- 1/2 cup applesauce, unsweetened
- 2 large eggs
- 2 cups carrots, shredded (6 medium carrots)
- 2-inch piece ginger, fresh (optional)

Nutrition Per Serving

Calories	206 cal
Protein	4 g
Sodium	135 mg
Phosphorus	98 mg
Potassium	142 mg

Directions
- Preheat the oven to 350 degrees F.
- Coat the muffin tins lightly with nonstick spray or oil.
- In a big bowl, mix the dry ingredients.
- Mix the wet ingredients in a medium-sized bowl using a fork or whisk.
- Stir the wet ingredients till just mixed into the dry ingredients.
- Combine with the carrots (shredded). Also, mix in as little as possible.
- Fill the muffins with the batter evenly.

- For 20 minutes, bake.

36. Chinese Sponge Cake

4 servings

Ingredients
- 1/2 cup sugar, granulated.
- 2 large eggs
- 1/4 tsp. baking powder
- 1/2 cup flour, all-purpose, sifted.
- 1/2 tsp. vanilla

Nutrition Per Serving

Calories	194 cal
Protein	5 g
Sodium	62 mg
Phosphorus	67 mg
Potassium	50 mg

Directions
- Preheat the oven to 325° F.
- By filling the pan halfway with the water, build a water bath; put it in the center of the oven rack to preheat.
- Line four custard cups or ramekins with parchment paper.
- Beat the eggs for 10 minutes on low.
- Gradually add the sugar while proceeding to beat the eggs.
- Stir in the vanilla.
- Mix the baking powder or flour and fold them into the egg mixture.
- Pour into the lined ramekins and put in a preheated oven in a water bath.
- Cook for at least 30 minutes until the tops are slightly browned, and a toothpick inserted in the middle comes out clean.

37. Chocolate Mint Cake

12 servings

Ingredients
- 2 cups sugar
- 2 cups flour, all-purpose
- 2 tsp. baking soda
- 4 oz. chocolate, unsweetened
- 1 stick butter, unsalted
- 1 tsp. low sodium baking powder

- 1 cup whipping cream, heavy
- 2 eggs
- 1 cup water
- 1 tsp. apple cider vinegar
- 2 tsp. peppermint extract
- 1 1/2 cups sour cream for frosting
- 1 1/2 cups chocolate chip, semisweet for frosting

Nutrition Per Serving

Calories	354 cal
Protein	5 g
Sodium	231 mg
Phosphorus	82 mg
Potassium	94 mg

Directions
- Preheat the oven to 375°. First, melt the chocolate, sugar, water, and butter over medium flame in a large saucepan. Stir occasionally till the ingredients are mixed well. Move to a large bowl and let cool.
- Add the baking soda, flour, and baking powder to a medium bowl. Combine the apple cider vinegar and cream in a small bowl and set it aside.
- While cooling the chocolate mixture, flour, and grease two 9' round cake pans with the butter. It is suggested to add a lining of parchment paper, as the cake is very soggy and can stick to the pans.
- To the melted chocolate, add the vinegar mixture and cream. Lightly mix, then add the eggs. Gently mix in the dry ingredients, taking care not to over-mix.
- Add mint extract and whisk gently after all the ingredients are well blended.
- Into the baking pans, add the cake batter. Bake for 30 to 35 minutes on the middle rack just till the inserted toothpick comes out clean.
- Before removing it from the baking pan, let it cool for at least 30 minutes.
- Make frosting when the cake is cooling. Melt the chocolate chips in a double boiler till smooth. Slowly add the sour cream till it's mixed well, after making the chocolate chill for a few minutes.
- When the cake is fully cooled, frost and serve!

38. Chocolate Mocha Cheesecake

8 servings

Ingredients
- 1/4 lb. unsalted butter
- 12 oz. chocolate wafer cookies

- 12 oz. cream cheese
- 1/4 cup of coffee liqueur
- 12 oz. chocolate chips
- 6 eggs
- 1/4 cup sugar
- 2 tsp. vanilla
- 1 cup of whipping cream, unwhipped

Nutrition Per Serving

Calories	537 cal
Protein	9 g
Sodium	280 mg
Phosphorus	52 mg
Dietary Fiber	34 g
Potassium	67 mg

Directions
- Preheat the oven to 350-degree.
- Crush the wafer cookies.
- Measure three cups of crumbs, then use a pastry blender to cut the butter.
- Push into the bottom and fill up to a springform pan that is 9" by 3".
- Refrigerate till it becomes firm.
- Over the simmering water, melt half of the chocolate. Let it cool.
- Beat until fluffy and light, the sugar, and the cream cheese; then add eggs and mix well.
- Mix well the cream, liqueur, melted chocolate, and vanilla.
- Remove the crust from the refrigerator and add the filling evenly.
- Put for an hour in the oven, and then confirm if the core is solid and do not jiggle when it is lightly shaken). If required, leave-in.
- Melt the leftover chocolate and pour it over the top. Before serving, let it cool to solidify.

39. Chocolate Orange Raisin Cookies

36 servings

Ingredients
- 3 cups flour, all-purpose
- 1 cup cocoa powder, unsweetened
- 1 tbsp. low sodium baking powder
- 1 1/3 cups of margarine
- 1/4 cup artificial sweetener, powdered.

- 4 eggs
- 2/3 cup of orange juice
- 2 cups raisins

Nutrition Per Serving

Calories	141 cal
Protein	2 g
Sodium	66 mg
Phosphorus	52 mg
Dietary Fiber	8 g
Potassium	139 mg

Directions
- Preheat the oven to 375°.
- Sift the cocoa, baking powder, and flour together.
- Beat the margarine till creamy by using a hand mixer or stand; mix in artificial sweetener.
- Add the eggs and stir well.
- Alternately with the orange juice, add the dry ingredients.
- Stir in the raisins.
- Drop teaspoonfuls of cookie dough on unbuttered baking sheets.
- For 10 minutes, bake.
- Remove and cool it down.

40. Dessert Pizza

8 servings

Ingredients
- 1/2-1 cup ricotta cheese, part-skim
- 2 cups fresh sliced strawberry or canned peaches
- 1/4-1/2 cup light-colored jam or apricot jam
- 5 tbsp. sugar, powdered, divided.
- 2 tbsp. warm jelly (or preserves)
- 1/4 cup of chocolate chips
- 1 - 12-inch pizza crust, precooked.

Nutrition Per Serving

Calories	288 cal
Protein	8 g
Sodium	166 mg
Phosphorus	47 mg
Potassium	98 mg

Directions
- Preheat the oven to 425°.
- Strain the ricotta with the cheesecloth or use a coffee filter.
- Drain the peaches in a colander and melt the jam for 30 seconds in the microwave.
- Brush the jam on the crust.
- Mix together the ricotta and 3 tbsp. of powdered sugar, spread on the crust.
- Sprinkle with the leftover chocolate chips and powdered sugar and top the ricotta with the strawberry or peach slices.
- For 10 to 12 minutes, bake.

41. Pie Crust

8 servings

Ingredients
- 2 tbsp. sugar
- 1 1/2 cups of flour
- 1/2 cup of vegetable oil
- 2 tbsp. milk

Nutrition Per Serving

Calories	219 cal
Protein	2 g
Sodium	2 mg
Phosphorus	29 mg
Dietary Fiber	14 g
Potassium	31 mg

Directions
- Pour the milk and oil together. Add to the flour and mix gently with a fork.
- Form it into a ball by using your hands.
- Roll in between two waxed paper pieces. Peel the top paper off and place the dough, paper side up, onto a pie plate when the dough is rolled out to around a 12-inch circle. Remove the top papers.
- Trim the crust with a fork about half an inch from the pan, fold the sides under, and flute the sides.
- Prick the sides and bottom of the baked pie shell and bake it at 450° for at least 12 minutes, just until it is golden brown.
- Fill with a pie filling for an unbaked shell and bake as instructed in the filling recipe.
- Makes one nine-inch pie shell.

42. Blueberry-Lemon Parfait

4 servings

Ingredients
- 10 crumbled gingersnaps
- 2 cartons (8 oz.) lemon yogurt
- 2 cups thawed frozen or fresh blueberries.

Nutrition Per Serving

Calories	220 cal
Protein	7 g
Sodium	137 mg
Phosphorus	182 mg
Potassium	361 mg

Directions
- Put 1/4 cup of blueberries in four wine glasses, mason jars, or bowls, followed by 1/4 cup of yogurt, next crumbled gingersnaps.
- To make two layers of each ingredient, repeat.

43. Fantastic Fudge

48 servings

Ingredients
- 4 (1 oz.) squares, chopped fine, unsweetened chocolate.
- 32 oz. chocolate chips, semisweet
- 2 cans (14 oz.) condensed milk, sweetened.
- 1 tsp. baking soda
- 2 cups walnuts
- 2 tbsp. vanilla

Nutrition Per Serving

Calories	190 cal
Protein	3 g
Sodium	62 mg
Phosphorus	94 mg
Dietary Fiber	11 g
Potassium	172 mg

Directions
- Line the bottom of a 9" by 13" pan with aluminum foil.
- Spray using a nonstick spray.
- Toss, in the top of the double boiler, the baking soda and chocolate till mixed well.

- Add in vanilla and condensed milk.
- Place at least 2 cups of boiling water over a double boiler pan.
- Stir with the spatula for 2 to 4 minutes before the chocolate is almost melted. There must remain a few tiny bits.
- Remove the pan from the flame and continue stirring for at least 2 minutes before the chocolate is completely melted and the mixture is smooth.
- Stir in the nuts.
- Transfer it to the pan.
- Till set, refrigerate for almost 2 hours.
- Remove the fudge from the pan.
- Slice into 48 (1 1/4 inch) squares.

44. Fried Apples

5 servings
Ingredients
- 2 tsp. cinnamon
- 5 cups sliced and peeled apples.
- 1 tsp. vanilla

Nutrition Per Serving

Calories	94 cal
Protein	0 g
Sodium	1 g
Phosphorus	10 mg
Potassium	153 mg

Directions
- Spray the skillet with the nonstick coating.
- Add the apples.
- Sauté the apples until they are soft.
- Add vanilla and cinnamon.

Chapter 6: Tasty Beverages and Snacks for Dialysis Diets

Are you craving sweet or savoury? Here are some tasty recipes for beverages and snacks that will always delight you. In search of anything easy? Our recipes for snacks will enable you to make healthy decisions.

1. Barbecue Turkey Wings

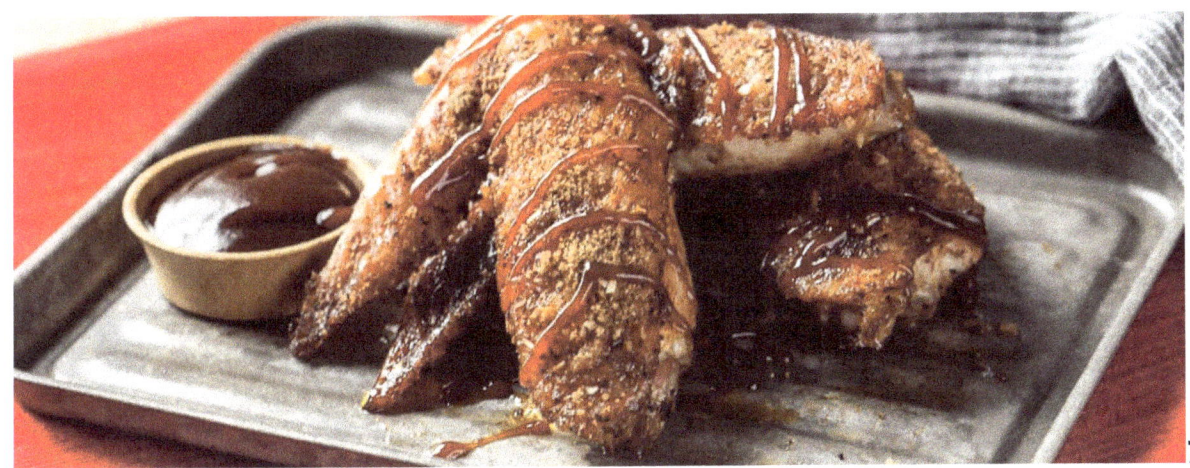

7 servings

Ingredients
- Chef McCargo's Spice Rub (Barbecue
- 7 whole turkey wings
- 2 tsp. onion flakes, dehydrated
- 1 tsp. black pepper
- 1 cup dark brown sugar, packed
- 2 tsp. granulated garlic
- 1 tsp. smoked paprika
- 2 tsp. dark chili powder
- 1 tsp. red pepper flakes
- 14 tbsp. low-sodium barbecue sauce (and 2 tbsp. per wing)

Nutrition Per Serving

Calories	272 cal
Protein	19 g
Sodium	371 mg
Phosphorus	155 mg
Dietary Fiber	0.6 g
Potassium	321 mg

Directions

- Preheat the oven to 375 °F.
- Pat the wings dry and pierce both sides with a fork.
- Rub the wings with spice rub liberally, saving 1 tbsp for later.
- Place the wings on the baking sheet and bake for 30 minutes, covered in foil. Remove the wings and discard the foil, turn over and cook for an extra 30 minutes. Sprinkle the remainder of the seasoning on the wings, then turn back over.
- Turn off the oven and let the wings stay for 15 minutes in the oven, then serve with reduced-sodium barbecue sauce on the side.

2. Chipotle Wings

4 servings (1 serving = 4 pieces)

Ingredients
- Oil for greasing the baking sheet tray
- 1 lb. jumbo chicken wings, fresh, slice in pieces or twenty individual pieces
- 1 tbsp. chopped chives
- ¼ cup honey
- 1½ tbsp. chipotle peppers, diced, in adobo sauce
- 1 tsp. black pepper
- ¼ cup unsalted, slightly melted butter

Nutrition Per Serving

Calories	384 cal
Protein	20 g
Sodium	99 mg
Phosphorus	146 mg
Dietary Fiber	0 g
Potassium	266 mg

Directions
- Preheat the oven to 400° F.
- On a wide nonstick greased baking sheet tray, put the precut wings.
- Bake for 18 to 20 minutes on an instant-read thermometer, flipping halfway through the cooking period or till crispy on the outside and hitting an internal temp. of 165 °F.
- In a large bowl, add remaining ingredients and mix with a spatula till well combined.
- Take out the wings from the oven and toss till evenly covered in the sauce. Transfer and serve on a large platter.

3. Cornbread Muffins and Citrus Honey Butter

12 muffins (1 serving = 1 muffin)
Ingredients
- 1 cup flour
- 1 cup cornmeal
- 3 tbsp. lemon juice
- 1 ½ tsp. baking soda
- 1 cup milk
- 1 beaten egg
- 1 tbsp. vanilla extract
- ½ stick, melted, and unsalted butter

Honey Butter:
- 1 stick softened, unsalted butter
- 2 tbsp. honey
- ½ tsp. orange extract
- ¼ tsp. black pepper
- ½ tsp. orange zest

Nutrition Per Serving

Calories	208 cal
Protein	3 g
Sodium	179 mg
Phosphorus	67 mg
Dietary Fiber	1 g
Potassium	87 mg

Directions
- Preheat the oven to 400° F.
- Beat the egg, butter, and milk together in a big bowl till well mixed.
- Mix the flour, baking soda, and cornmeal in a separate bowl, then fold into the liquid ingredients till smooth. Be careful not to overbeat.
- Line the muffin tins with the liner, then fill each cup ¾ full, and bake on the center rack for 15 to 20 minutes.
- Whisk the honey butter ingredients in a small bowl until mixed; scatter on the top of the cornbread muffins or serve on the side.

4. Chocolate Smoothie

4 servings (1 serving = 6 oz. glass)
Ingredients

- 2 cups ice
- 2 scoops of chocolate-flavored whey protein
- ¼ cup condensed milk
- ½ cup evaporated milk
- Pinch of nutmeg
- ¼ tsp. ground cinnamon
- Optional: 2 tbsp. Southern Comfort liqueur

Nutrition Per Serving

Calories	142 cal
Protein	10 g
Sodium	134 mg
Phosphorus	162 mg
Dietary Fiber	0.9 g
Potassium	247 mg

Directions
- Mix all the ingredients in a blender, excluding cinnamon on high till smooth, for almost 1 to 2 minutes.
- To garnish, sprinkle with cinnamon or top with whipped cream.

5. Cucumber Cups with Buffalo Chicken Salad

8 servings (1 serving = about 2 to 3 oz.)

Ingredients
- 1 tsp. Smoked paprika
- ½ tsp. black pepper
- 1 tsp. Cayenne pepper
- ½ tsp. Italian seasoning
- ½ cup of Kraft mayonnaise
- 2 tbsp. hot sauce
- 2 tbsp. lemon juice
- 1 tbsp. chopped fresh garlic
- ¼ cup of blue cheese crumbs
- 3 cups shredded or diced chicken breast
- 2 tbsp. chopped, fresh chives
- For garnish: ¼ cup fresh, chopped parsley.
- 2 seedless, large cucumbers, diced into 1-inch slices, with their centers (half of them) scooped out (15 to 20 slices)

Nutrition Per Serving

| Calories | 155 cal |

Protein	18 g
Sodium	252 mg
Phosphorus	189 mg
Dietary Fiber	0.6 g
Potassium	283 mg

Directions

- In a medium-size bowl, mix all the ingredients, excluding the cucumbers and chicken.
- Stir in the chicken and stir till thoroughly coated. Put aside for about 30 minutes in the refrigerator.
- Remove from the refrigerator, spoon equal quantities (about 1 to 2 tsp.) onto each slice of cucumber. Garnish with parsley.

6. Cauliflower Phyllo Cups

24 cups (1 serving = 1 phyllo cup)

Ingredients

- ½ cup shredded Swiss cheese, reduced-sodium
- 3 beaten eggs, lightly scrambled
- 2 tbsp. butter
- ½ cup shredded cheddar cheese
- 1½ cups diced cauliflower drained and cooked
- 4 slices uncured and natural bacon, diced
- 2 tbsp. diced jalapeños
- ¼ cup finely diced onions
- 1 tbsp. parsley
- ½ tsp. red pepper flakes
- 3 sheets phyllo dough
- ½ tsp. ground black pepper
- Optional garnish: ground black pepper and parsley

Nutrition Per Serving

Calories	68 cal
Protein	3 g
Sodium	107 mg
Phosphorus	49 mg
Dietary Fiber	0.3 g
Potassium	42 mg

Directions

- Preheat the oven to 375 ° F.

- Lightly scramble the eggs in a large sauté pan, take them off from the pan, and put them aside.
- Melt the butter in the same pan. Sauté the bacon before it's cooked. Add the onions, jalapeños, flakes of red pepper, and cauliflower and sauté till the onions are translucent. Use ground black pepper and parsley to season.
- Remove from the flame and whisk in 2 cheeses and scrambled eggs.
- Layer the three Phyllo Sheets.
- Cut the sheets into 24 squares and place them into a muffin tin pan, slightly sprayed.
- Load per muffin cup with equal quantities of mixture and bake for 12 to 15 minutes on the oven's bottom shelf or till moderately golden around the edges. Turn the oven off and leave to rest for 2 to 3 minutes.
- Optional: Use ground black pepper and parsley to garnish.

7. Sweet and Nutty Protein Bars

12 serving (1 serving = 2 oz. bar)
Ingredients
- ½ cup almonds
- 2½ cups toasted and rolled oats
- ½ cup peanut butter
- ½ cup flaxseeds
- ½ cup honey
- 1 cup dried blueberries, craisins, or cherries

Nutrition Per Serving

Calories	283 cal
Protein	7 g
Sodium	49 mg
Phosphorus	177 mg
Dietary Fiber	5.8 g
Potassium	258 mg

Directions
- For 10 minutes or till golden brown, toast the oats by putting the rolled oats on the baking sheet in a 350 °F oven.
- Combine all the ingredients till mixed well.
- In a lightly greased 9" x 9" pan, push the protein mix down. For at least 1 hour or overnight, wrap and refrigerate.
- Slice the bars of protein into the required squares and serve.

8. Herbed Biscuits

12 servings (1 serving = 1 biscuit)

Ingredients
- 1 tsp. cream of tartar
- 1¾ cups flour, all-purpose
- nonstick cooking spray
- ¼ cup mayonnaise
- ½ tsp. baking soda
- 3 tbsp. chives or another herb (fresh or dry to taste)
- ⅔ cup skim milk

Nutrition Per Serving

Calories	109 cal
Protein	3 g
Sodium	88 mg
Phosphorus	34 mg
Dietary Fiber	1 g
Potassium	85 mg

Directions
- Preheat the oven to 400° F. Next, brush the non-stick cooking spray on a cookie sheet.
- Combine the tartar cream, baking soda, and flour in a large bowl. Then stir with a fork after adding mayonnaise, so the mixture appears like coarse cornmeal.
- Combine the herbs and milk in a tiny bowl and add them to the mixture of flour till well mixed; keep stirring.
- Place the heaping tbsp. on cookie sheet. For 10 minutes, bake.
- Till ready to use, refrigerate.

9. Heavenly Deviled Eggs

4 servings (1 serving = 2 halves)

Ingredients
- 2 tbsp. light mayonnaise
- 4 eggs, large, boiled hard with the shells removed
- ¼ tsp. Ground black pepper
- ½ tsp. Cider vinegar
- ½ tsp. dry mustard
- 1 tbsp. finely chopped onion
- Dash of paprika for garnish

Nutrition Per Serving

Calories	98 cal
Protein	6 g
Sodium	124 mg
Phosphorus	90 mg
Dietary Fiber	0 g
Potassium	73 mg

Directions

- Slice the eggs lengthwise in two. Remove the yolks carefully and put them in a tiny bowl. Put the egg white on the plate.
- Mash the yolks with a fork and add the vinegar, dry mustard, onion, and black pepper to the mixture.
- Refill the cooked egg white with the yolk mixture, piling gently.
- Optional: Sprinkle the deviled eggs with the paprika and serve.

10. 60-Sec Salsa

8 SERVINGS

Ingredients

- 2 chopped green onions
- 4 chopped plum or Roma tomatoes
- 1/2 - 1 chopped green bell pepper
- 3 minced garlic cloves
- 1/2 bunch fresh chopped cilantro
- 1/2 - 1 fresh, chopped jalapeño
- 1/4 cup fresh chopped oregano, or 1 tbsp. dried
- 1/2 tsp. cumin

Nutrition Per Serving

Calories	14 cal
Protein	1 g
Sodium	4 mg
Phosphorus	14 mg
Dietary Fiber	0 g
Potassium	117 mg

Directions

- In a blender or a food processor, combine all ingredients till the larger pieces are chunky and small.
- Let it remain in the refrigerator for a few hours.
- Best served with simple tortilla chips and chilled.

11. Alfredo Sauce

8 servings

Ingredients
- 3 tbsp. flour, all-purpose
- 1/4 cup olive oil
- 2 cups rice milk
- 1 minced clove garlic
- 1/3 cup Parmesan cheese, shredded
- 4 oz. cream cheese
- 1 tbsp. lemon juice
- 1/4 tsp. ground nutmeg

Nutrition Per Serving

Calories	173 cal
Protein	3 g
Sodium	142 mg
Phosphorus	75 mg
Potassium	32 mg

Directions
- Over a medium flame, heat the olive oil in a skillet. To prepare a paste, add the flour and whisk, then mix in minced garlic.
- Add the rice milk slowly, frequently whisking to avoid lumps. Let the mixture boil and let it thicken.
- Add the cream cheese and blend thoroughly. Remove from the flame.
- Add 1/3 cup of Parmesan cheese, lemon juice, and nutmeg. Mix thoroughly.
- Serve over chicken, pasta, or steamed vegetables, etc.

12. Apple Cup Cider

8 SERVINGS

Ingredients
- 2 cinnamon sticks
- 2 quarts apple juice, 100%
- 1 pinch nutmeg
- 1/2 tsp. cloves, whole
- 1 tsp. allspice

Nutrition Per Serving

Calories	114 cal
Protein	0 g

Sodium	28 mg
Phosphorus	1 mg
Dietary Fiber	0 g
Potassium	255 mg

Directions
- In a large saucepan, pour the apple juice and proceed to heat over medium-high flame.
- Add the remaining ingredients.
- Boil, then reduce to low heat. For 10 minutes, let "steep."
- Pour the cider into a thermos or a mug using a fine metal sieve when ready to serve.

13. Beef Jerky

30 SERVINGS

Ingredients
- 3 lb. flank steak or lean meat
- 3/4 cup soy sauce, reduced-sodium (lite)
- 1/2 cup red wine
- 1/4 cup of dark brown sugar
- 2 tbsp. liquid smoke
- 1 1/2 tsp. Worcestershire sauce
- 2-3 drops of Tabasco sauce
- 1 tsp. garlic powder
- 1 tsp. liquid pepper sauce

Nutrition Per Serving
Calories	100 cal
Protein	12 g
Sodium	100 mg
Phosphorus	190 mg
Potassium	100 mg

Directions
- Trim all the fat from a 3 lb. lean meat or flank steak.
- Cut into 30 long strips, lengthwise, with the grain.
- In a glass dish, put the strips.
- Mix with all the remaining ingredients and spill over the beef.
- For almost 5 hours or overnight, cover and refrigerate.
- Remove from the marinade till you are about to dry the meat.
- Set it to 145° and dry the meat for 5 to 20 hours, if you've a dehydrator.
- Preheat to 175° if you're using the oven.

- On top of the baking sheets, place the wire racks and lay the strips, so they do not overlap.
- For 10 to 12 hours, bake. The beef jerky, when done, must be dry and brittle.
- Store the jerky in a plastic bag or container that is airtight. If it lasts more than a week, put it in the fridge.

14. Brown Bag Popcorn

1 SERVING

Ingredients
- 1 tsp. canola oil
- 1/4 cup popcorn kernels
- 1 brown paper lunch bag

Nutrition Per Serving

Calories	155 cal
Protein	4 g
Sodium	0 mg
Phosphorus	96 mg
Dietary Fiber	4 g
Potassium	105 mg

Directions
- Mix the oil and popcorn together in a small bowl.
- In a brown bag, place the popcorn, fold to close it and staple twice the top.
- Microwave for 3 minutes on maximum or just till there's 5 seconds between the pops.

15. Dilled Cream-Cheese Spread

8 servings

Ingredients
- 1 tsp. onion powder
- 8 oz. whipped cream cheese
- 1/2 tsp. chopped fresh dill

Nutrition Per Serving

Calories	70 cal
Protein	1 g
Sodium	59 mg
Phosphorus	22 mg
Potassium	26 mg

Directions
- Mix together all the ingredients with the electric mixer.
- Store in a container that is airtight in the refrigerator.

16. Fruit Salsa

4 servings

Ingredients
- 3/4 cup diced mango
- 3/4 cup diced pineapple
- 1/4 cup diced red onion
- 1/2 cup diced strawberries
- 2 tbsp. chopped, fresh mint leaves
- 1 jalapeño, seeded, stemmed, and finely diced
- 1 tbsp. lime juice
- 2 tbsp. orange juice

Nutrition Per Serving

Calories	59 cal
Protein	1 g
Sodium	9 mg
Phosphorus	16 mg
Potassium	155 mg

Directions
- In a glass bowl or medium ceramic, mix all the ingredients together and stir well to blend.
- Before serving, cover with plastic wrap and let the salsa marinate for at least 20 to 30 minutes.

17. Ginger Cranberry Punch

4 servings

Ingredients
- 1/2 cup fresh peeled ginger, sliced thin
- 4 cups cranberry juice
- 1/3 cup sugar, granulated
- 1/3 cup lime juice, fresh

Nutrition Per Serving

Calories	124 cal
Protein	0 g

Sodium	0 mg
Phosphorus	1 mg
Potassium	50 mg

Directions
- Bring the ginger and the juice to a boil in a large pan.
- Cook it over a medium flame to infuse the flavor for at least 20 minutes.
- Add the sugar and the lime juice, whisk until dissolved.
- Strain and then serve.

18. Green Tomatillo Salsa

2 tbsp. servings per recipe

Ingredients
- 1 diced onion
- 1 lb. tomatillos
- 3 tbsp. lime juice
- 1 each jalapeño
- 1 each garlic cloves
- 1/2 cup cilantro
- 1 tbsp. olive oil

Nutrition Per Serving

Calories	20 cal
Protein	0 g
Sodium	6 mg
Phosphorus	10 mg
Potassium	86 mg

Directions
- Remove husks from the tomatillos and clean off the sticky or oily residue on the skin.
- Toss the tomatillos, cloves of garlic, some olive oil with the jalapeño, and onion.
- Roast till soft and a little charred, at 400 degrees F.
- Let it cool.
- Add the lime juice and cilantro.
- Combine the ingredients till well mixed in a food processor or a blender.
- Salsa is kept fresh in the fridge for 2 weeks or in the freezer for up to 6 months.

19. Green Tomatoes and Goat Cheese

4 servings

Ingredients
- 1 tbsp. balsamic vinegar

- 8 slices of French bread, toasted
- 4 green tomatoes, medium
- 1 cup crumbled goat cheese
- 2 tsp. minced oregano leaves
- ground pepper to taste
- 4 tsp. olive oil

Nutrition Per Serving

Calories	173 cal
Protein	7 g
Sodium	135 mg
Phosphorus	161 mg
Potassium	280 mg

Directions
- Slice the tomatoes into thick 1/2-inch slices.
- Use oil to spray on a shallow baking dish.
- Put the tomato slices in the bottom of the dish, in an overlapping, single layer.
- Sprinkle the vinegar on the tomatoes and spread the oregano over the tomatoes.
- Top with the goat's crumbled cheese, and drizzle with the olive oil.
- Broil 5 to 8 inches under a preheated broiler and broil for around 7 to 8 minutes before the tomatoes are hot and the cheese is just beginning to brown.
- Put on the toasted bread, and season with the pepper.
- Serve immediately.

Chapter 7: Side Dishes

1. BBQ Asparagus

6 Servings

Ingredients
- 2-3 tbsp. extra-virgin olive oil
- 1/2 lb. fresh Asparagus (12 to 15 large spears)
- 2-3 tbsp. lemon juice
- 1/2 tsp. pepper

Nutrition Per Serving

Calories	86 kcals
Protein	3 g
Sodium	4 mg
Phosphorus	41 mg
Dietary Fiber	2 g
Potassium	196 mg

Directions
- In a shallow dish large enough for rolling the asparagus into it, mix the oil, lemon juice, and black pepper and cover fully with the mixture.
- Wash & trim the asparagus spears woody ends.
- Put in the oil mixture and leave the asparagus in the bowl. To prevent the oil from dripping, put the tray on a dish in the refrigerator to marinate till the grill is prepared.
- Prepare the gas or charcoal barbecue and heat the med-high heat.
- To prevent the spears from pan sticking, gently spray the vegetable grilling tray, a sheet or grill basket of tin foil folded heavy-duty into a tray with olive oil spray.
- On a vegetable grilling tray, place the asparagus and pour the leftover oil onto the spears from the dish.
- Grill the asparagus until tender and start browning, regularly rotating, around 5 mins, on the tin foil or in the pan. Move to plate. Serve at room temperature or warm.

2. BBQ Corn on the Cob

8 Servings

Ingredients
- 1 tbs. grated parmesan cheese

- 3 tbsps. olive oil
- 1 tsp. parsley
- 1 tsp. dried thyme
- 4 fresh corn on the cob, in 8 halves
- 1/2 tsp. black pepper

Nutrition Per Serving

Calories	109 kcals
Protein	2 g
Sodium	15 mg
Phosphorus	59 mg
Dietary Fiber	2 g
Potassium	189 mg

Directions

- Husk & clean the corn.
- Mix oil, cheese, parsley, thyme, and black pepper in a wide enough to put the corn into it and fully cover with mixture.
- In the mixture, place the corn and roll to coat the corn thoroughly.
- Place all the corn in mid of an aluminum foil sheet (heavy-duty).
- Fold the edges of the foil sheet for creating a tray making sure not to leave space for the oil to drip onto the grill.
- On the grill, place the foil tray over med heat and cook for 15-20 mins turning as browning on each side.

3. Low Salt Macaroni and Cheese

4 Servings

Ingredients

- 2 to 3 cups of boiling water
- 1/4 tsp dried mustard
- 2 cups of noodles (any shape)
- 1 tsp margarine/salt-free butter
- 1/2 cup of grated cheddar cheese

Nutrition Per Serving

| Calories | 163 kcals |
| Protein | 6 g |

Sodium	114 mg
Phosphorus	138 mg
Dietary Fiber	3 g
Potassium	39 mg

Directions
- Boil water, then adds noodles, & cook for about 5-7 mins till tender.
- Drain it.
- While very hot, sprinkle it with cheese, then stir in butter & mustard.

4. Grilled Vegetables

Grilled vegetables are more flavorful and tastier. Grilled vegetables bring variety to your everyday meal. So, take your cooking skills outdoor and get grilling

Asparagus 1/2 cup (6 spears)
- 49 mg. Phosphorus
- 202 mg potassium
- 13 mg sodium

Carrots ½ Cup
- 23mg phosphorus
- 183 mg potassium
- 5 mg sodium

Cucumber ½ Cup
- 12mg phosphorus
- 76 mg potassium
- 1 mg sodium

Eggplant 1 Cup
- 15mg phosphorus
- 122mg potassium
- 1 mg sodium

Green Pepper 1 Small
- 15mg phosphorus
- 130mg potassium
- 2 mg sodium

Mushrooms 1 Cup
- 30 mg phosphorus

- 111 mg potassium
- 2 mg sodium

5. Cool Coconut Marshmallow Salad

8 Servings

Ingredients

- 1 cup of dried coconut, shredded.
- 8.8 oz. (1 package) fruit-flavored marshmallows
- 2 cups of sour cream
- 1 can (15 ounces) of drained fruit cocktail

Nutrition Per Serving

Calories	317 kcals
Protein	3 g
Sodium	48 mg
Phosphorus	74 mg
Dietary Fiber	3 g
Potassium	185 mg

Directions

- In a bowl, mix all the ingredients.
- To serve, move to a glass bowl.
- If you want a creamy salad, before serving, refrigerate for an hour & refrigerate overnight, if you want a molded salad.

6. Cauliflower in Mustard Sauce

4 Servings

Ingredients

- 1 tsp. honey
- 2 tsps. Dijon mustard
- 1 tbsp olive oil
- 1 tbsp + 2 tsps. white wine vinegar
- Dash black pepper.
- 2 cups of cauliflower flowerets

Calories	51 kcals
Protein	1 g
Sodium	75 mg

Phosphorus	25 mg
Dietary Fiber	1 g
Potassium	163 mg

Directions

- Whisk together the mustard & honey; whisk in the vinegar & then the olive oil.
- Season with black pepper. Then Set aside.
- To boiling water, add the cauliflower & cook till tender.
- Drain it well.
- With the dressing, toss the drained & cooked cauliflower.
- For 30-45 mins, allow it to cool & serve.

7. Pineapple Coleslaw

4 Servings

Ingredients

- 1 (8 oz) can of crushed, drained unsweetened pineapple
- Dash of pepper (optional)
- 2 cups of shredded cabbage
- 1/4 cup of chopped onion
- 1/4 cup of Miracle Whip

Nutrition Per Serving

Calories	72 kcals
Protein	1 g
Sodium	137 mg
Phosphorus	15 mg
Dietary Fiber	1 g
Potassium	153 mg

Directions

- Mix all the ingredients together.
- before serving, chill for 1 hour at least

8. Acorn Squash Baked with Pineapple

2 Servings

Ingredients

- 1 acorn squash, cut in half, & seeded.
- 1/4 tsp. nutmeg

- 2 tsps. + 1 tbsp unsalted butter
- 3 tbsps. pineapple, crushed.
- 2 tsps. brown sugar

Nutrition Per Serving

Calories	202 kcals
Protein	2 g
Sodium	90 mg
Phosphorus	80 mg
Potassium	783 mg

Directions
- Preheat the oven to 400°F.
- In a greased baking pan, place the squash with the cut side up.
- In each Acorn half, put one tsp of butter + one tsp of brown sugar.
- With aluminum foil, cover the squash & bake for around 30 mins until tender.
- Scoop cooked squash from the shells, leaving the shell 1/4" thick.
- Combine the cooked squash, 1 tbsp of butter, pineapple & nutmeg. Beat until smooth.
- Spoon the mixture into the shells; heat for around 15 mins at 425 degrees F.

9. Apple & Cherry Chutney

32 (1 TBSP EACH) SERVINGS

Ingredients
- 1 cup of dried tart cherries
- 1 med. tart apple
- 1 1/2 cups of sugar
- 1 cup of apple cider vinegar
- 1 thinly sliced small red onion.

Nutrition Per Serving

Calories	55 kcals
Protein	1 g
Sodium	2 mg
Phosphorus	1 mg
Potassium	12 mg

Directions
- Cut the apple into thin slices, keeping the skin on.
- With the onions, sugar, & vinegar, put the apples & cherries in a large saucepan. Cook and whisk before the sugar has dissolved and started boiling the mixture.

- Cover & decrease the heat to low & simmer for around 8-10 mins, till the onions are tender & plump & tender is the dried cherries.
- Uncover and raise the heat to full and boil till the syrup is reduced to a glossy glaze around the fruit, around 5 more mins. Chutney can be served at once or held for many days, covered & refrigerated.

10. Asian Pear Salad

4 SERVINGS

Ingredients
- 1/2 cup of water
- 1/2 cup of sugar
- 6 cups of green leaf lettuce
- 1/2 cup of walnuts or pecans
- 2 ounces blue cheese or stilton
- 4 Asian pears, cored, peeled, and diced.
- serve with oil & vinegar dressing.
- 1/2 cup of pomegranate seeds

Nutrition Per Serving

Calories	301 kcals
Protein	6 g
Sodium	206 mg
Phosphorus	127 mg
Dietary Fiber	14 g
Potassium	297 mg

Directions
- In a non-stick pan, dissolve the sugar & water.
- Heat until it forms a syrup.
- Stir in the nuts quickly.
- Turn out while still hot on parchment paper/aluminum foil & separate nuts. Let it cool.
- In a large bowl, put the lettuce.
- To lettuce, add pears, cheese, & pomegranate seeds.
- Sprinkle with nuts & serve with a dressing of oil and vinegar.
- Add the diced chicken breast to make this a full meal & make the serving a little bigger.

11. Basil Oil

16 SERVINGS

Ingredients
- 1 cup of vegetable oil or olive oil
- 1 1/2 cups of fresh basil leaves

Nutrition Per Serving

Calories	135 kcals
Protein	0 g
Sodium	0 mg
Phosphorus	0 mg
Dietary Fiber	15 g
Potassium	5 mg

Directions
- Drain 1 1/2 cups of lightly packed basil leaves and rinse.
- Pat leaves & dry with a towel.
- Stir together the basil leaves & 1 cup of olive or vegetable oil in a blender/ food processor. Just whirl until the leaves are chopped finely (don't puree).
- Pour the mixture over med heat into a 1 - 1 1/2-quart plate. Stir periodically before oil bubbles along the edges of the pan and hits 165 degrees F, 3-4 mins. To eliminate any mixture bacteria, make sure it is heated to this temp.
- Remove from heat & allow stand for around an hour until it cools.
- Line a fine wire strainer set over a wide bowl with 2 layers of cheesecloth.
- Pour a mixture of oil into a strainer.
- Gently press the basil onto the remaining oil after the oil passes through.
- Discard the basil.
- Serve the oil or hold it in the refrigerator in some airtight container for up to 3 months. When chilled, the olive oil will solidify somewhat, but when it gets back to room temp, it will liquefy rapidly.

12. BBQ Rub For Pork or Chicken

4 servings

Ingredients
- 1 tsp. smoked paprika.
- 1 tbsp. brown sugar
- 1 tsp. granulated garlic
- 1 tsp. chili powder
- Optional 1/8 tsp ground red pepper
- 1 tsp. cumin

- 1 tsp. onion powder
- 1/8 tsp. all spice
- 1/4 tsp. dry mustard powder

Nutrition Per Serving

Calories	20 kcals
Protein	0 g
Sodium	9 mg
Phosphorus	7 mg
Dietary Fiber	0 g
Potassium	34 mg

Directions
- In a bowl, mix together all the ingredients thoroughly.
- Rub on chicken or pork before cooking.

13. BBQ Winter Squash

8 servings

Ingredients
- 1-2 tbsps. olive oil
- 1-2 butternut squash or acorn sliced in 1-inch-thick slices.
- 1-2 tbsps. Butter
- 1-2 tbsps. brown sugar

Nutrition Per Serving

Calories	99 kcals
Protein	1 g
Sodium	3 mg
Phosphorus	53 mg
Dietary Fiber	6 g
Potassium	508 mg

Directions
- Heat grill to about 400 degrees F.
- Brush the squash with olive oil light coating and place it on the grill for about 5 mins, then turn.
- When the fork-tender, brush it with melted butter & brown sugar.
- Leave for 1 min on the grill, remove & serve.

14. Beet Salad

4 Servings

Ingredients
- 1/2 cup of pecans or walnuts
- 4, chilled beets, peeled, roasted, & diced.
- 2-3 ounces blue cheese or stilton.
- 1/4 cup of chopped fine fresh basil.
- 1 bed of leaf lettuce (per person)
- 2 tbsps. olive oil
- 1/2 cup of fruit/herb vinegar

Nutrition Per Serving

Calories	283 kcals
Protein	6 g
Sodium	241 mg
Phosphorus	102 mg
Dietary Fiber	2 g
Potassium	393 mg

Directions
- Heat the oven to 400°F.
- Roast beets till soft, 45 min. Approx.
- Chill, peel & dice.
- In a saucepan, incorporate the nuts, sugar & water. Heat the mixture, stirring continually until most of the liquid bubbles are gone.
- Pour nuts on parchment paper/aluminum foil when the nuts are covered & the frying pan is nearly dry, and separate nuts when still hot.
- Let it cool, and it can be kept for many months at room temp.
- Prepare a bed of lettuce.
- Toss the beets with basil, vinegar & oil.
- Sprinkle it on a plate of lettuce.
- Scatter all over the top of cheese cubes & nuts.

15. Berry Wild Rice Salad

8 Servings

Ingredients
- 2 cups of water
- 1 cup of uncooked wild rice
- 1/2 cup of chopped onion
- 1 cup of lightly steamed collard greens
- 1/4 cup of blueberries
- 2 1/2 cups of mixed berries (blackberry, raspberry, etc.)

- 1/4 cup of fresh mint, chopped.
- 2 tbsps. lemon juice
- 1/2 cup reduced-fat/fat-free sour cream.
- 1 tbsp. olive oil

Nutrition Per Serving

Calories	155 kcals
Protein	5 g
Sodium	21 mg
Phosphorus	98 mg
Dietary Fiber	2 g
Potassium	214 mg

Directions
- Put the water and rice in a wide saucepan.
- Carry to a boil, decrease the heat to low, then cover and simmer for 45-55 mins or till most of the liquid has been absorbed.
- Empty the rice and add the steamed greens, onions, and berries to a wide mixing bowl.
- Mix thoroughly.
- Purée all dressing ingredients, excluding sour cream in a blender/food processor until it is well mixed, incorporating more liquid if required.
- Whisk the sour cream slowly until well combined.
- Pour dressing over the rice salad and coat it.
- Serve promptly or place for later usage covered in the refrigerator.

16. Black-Eyed Peas

12 Servings

Ingredients
- 3 1/2 cups water/vegetable stock (low sodium).
- 2 cups of dried Black-eyed peas.
- 1 finely chopped med. Onion
- 12 ounces optional smoked turkey
- 1 cup diced celery.
- 5 - 6 finely chopped cloves garlic
- 1/2 tsp. ginger
- 1/2 tsp. thyme
- 1 pinch of cayenne pepper
- 1/2 tsp. curry powder

Nutrition Per Serving

Calories	130 kcals
Protein	12 g
Sodium	274 mg
Phosphorus	200 mg
Dietary Fiber	1 g
Potassium	434 mg

Directions
- In a big bowl, add black-eyed peas, then add water for covering it about 4 ". Cover and leave to soak for a minimum of 6 hrs. or overnight.
- Drain the peas under cool water and rinse.
- Add the black-eyed peas and the remaining ingredients to a large pot.
- Bring to boil, then decrease the heat to low, & cover with the lid and cook for around 1 1/2 hours till the peas are tender.
- Occasionally stir.

17. Blasted Brussels Sprouts

4-6 Servings
Ingredients
- 1-2 tbsps. olive oil
- 2 cups of Brussels Sprouts (around one stalk)
- 1/4 cup of fruit/herb-flavored vinegar
- 2-4 tbsps. Parmesan Cheese fresh grated

Nutrition Per Serving
Calories	68 kcals
Protein	3 g
Sodium	70 mg
Phosphorus	59 mg
Dietary Fiber	5 g
Potassium	182 mg

Directions
- To 450 degrees F, preheat the oven.
- With olive oil, toss the sprouts.
- Put it on a slightly oiled baking sheet.
- Roast for about 10 mins. When tender, sprouts are done.
- Now remove from the oven. Then Sprinkle with freshly grated Parmesan cheese & fruit vinegar.

18. Buttermilk Herb Ranch Dressing

2 tbsps. servings

Ingredients
- 1/2 cup of. of milk
- 1/4 tsp. garlic powder
- 1/2 cup of mayonnaise
- 1 tbsp. fresh chives, chopped.
- 2 tbsps. vinegar
- 1 tbsp. chopped oregano leaves.
- 1 tbsp. dill

Nutrition Per Serving

Calories	83 kcals
Protein	1 g
Sodium	64 mg
Phosphorus	1 mg
Potassium	9 mg

Directions
- In a med bowl, whisk milk, mayonnaise, & vinegar.
- Then add dill, fresh chives, & oregano leaves with garlic powder (1/4 tsp).
- Mix them together.
- Chill one hour at least to allow the flavors to develop.
- Before serving, stir dressing well.

19. Cajun Seasoning

2 SERVINGS

Ingredients
- 2 tsps. onion powder
- 2 tsps. paprika
- 1 tsp. cayenne for mild or 2 tsps. of for med. Spice
- 2 tsps. garlic powder

Nutrition Per Serving

Calories	25 kcals
Protein	1 g
Sodium	15 mg
Phosphorus	5 mg
Dietary Fiber	1 g
Potassium	36 mg

Directions

- Mix all of the ingredients together & store them in a container (airtight).

20. Chinese Five-Spice Blend

22 Servings

Ingredients

- 2 tbsps. ground cinnamon
- 1 tsp. anise seed
- 1/4 cup of ginger
- 1 tsp. ground allspice
- 2 tsps. ground cloves

Nutrition Per Serving

Calories	20 kcals
Protein	0 g
Sodium	14 mg
Phosphorus	4 mg
Dietary Fiber	1 g
Potassium	49 mg

Directions

- Mix all the ingredients together & store in a container (airtight).
- For one year, Ground spices are good, and for 2 years, whole spices are good.

21. Citrus Relish

8-12 Servings

Ingredients

- 1 quart of white vinegar
- 2-4 tbsps. Sugar
- 2 lbs. small lemons, kumquats, limes, or oranges
- glass jars
- 1/4 cup of mustard seed

Nutrition Per Serving

Calories	26 kcals
Protein	0 g
Sodium	0 mg
Phosphorus	4 mg

| Potassium | 37 mg |

Directions

Pickled Fruit

- For each fruit, cut a cross at the end of the stem. Quarter when using oranges.
- Put them in glass jars & cover them with vinegar.
- Add 2 tsps. of the mustard seed to every jar. Put lids on.
- Leave for around one month at room temp, then turn it into relish below & serve.

Citrus Relish

- With sugar, mix the fruit in a small frying pan and add more sugar, if required.
- Shake the pan regularly over med heat for 5-10 mins until the mixture cooks, and the fruit becomes glossy and translucent.
- Serve warm or cold.
- In salad dressing or for marinating chicken or fish, the remaining vinegar from pickled fruit could be used.

22. Coleslaw with a Kick

10 Servings

Ingredients

- 1 tbsp. Horseradish
- 1 cup of mayonnaise
- 3 tbsps. granulated sugar
- 2 tsps. cider vinegar
- 1 (1 lb.) bag coleslaw mix with carrots.
- 2 tsps. chopped fresh dill.

Nutrition Per Serving

Calories	107 kcals
Protein	0 g
Sodium	170 mg
Phosphorus	11 mg
Potassium	117 mg

Directions

- In a bowl, mix the mayonnaise, vinegar, sugar, horseradish, and dill together.
- Stir in the coleslaw mix till well blended.
- Chill for at least 1 hr. It will taste good if chilled overnight.

23. Collard Greens

4 Servings

Ingredients
- ½ chopped onion.
- 1 1/2 tsps. olive oil
- 1 large bunch stems removed collard greens.
- 2 tsps. minced garlic
- 1/2 tsp. red pepper flakes
- 1/8 tsp. black pepper
- tbsps. Vinegar
- 1/2 cups low-sodium, chicken broth fat free

Nutrition Per Serving

Calories	50 kcals
Protein	3 g
Sodium	40 mg
Phosphorus	34 mg
Dietary Fiber	2 g
Potassium	190 mg

Directions
- Over med heat, heat the oil, add the onions, and garlic & cook until soft (don't burn).
- Add greens (1/4), then toss in the garlic and onions.
- When the greens are wilted, incorporate the remaining greens until they are both added and wilted in batches.
- Add in the flakes of black pepper & red pepper.
- Stir in the broth and get it to a boil.
- Reduce the heat and simmer till tender or for 20 mins. It can almost absolutely reduce the broth.
- Remove from the heat and sprinkle before serving with vinegar.

24. Cornbread Muffins

12 Servings
Ingredients
- 1 cup of cornmeal
- 1 cup of all-purpose flour
- 1/4 cup of granulated sugar
- 1/2 cup canned corn (no salt added)
- 1/2 tsp. baking soda
- 2 eggs
- 1/2 cup softened unsalted butter.

- 1/2 cup of buttermilk
- 1/4 cup of honey

Nutrition Per Serving

Calories	203 kcals
Protein	4 g
Sodium	79 mg
Phosphorus	67 mg
Potassium	89 mg

Directions

- Preheat the oven to 400°C.
- To lightly grease the muffin pan, use a cooking oil spray.
- Combine the flour, baking soda, cornmeal, and sugar in a wide bowl.
- Using a pastry blender to mix in the butter or mix in the food processor until the butter is pea sized.
- Beat the eggs in a separate bowl.
- Add the buttermilk and honey.
- Pour the mixture of eggs into the mixture of flour, stirring till just mixed.
- Fold the corn up.
- Bake for 20-25 mins till a toothpick inserted in the middle of the muffin comes out clean. Spoon batter into the muffin cups.

25. Cornichon Pickles, Low Salt

24 Servings

Ingredients

- 4 sprigs of fresh tarragon
- 3 cups of cornichon/pickling cucumbers
- 1/2 tsp mustard seeds
- 1 tbsp kosher salt

Nutrition Per Serving

Calories	6 kcals
Protein	0 g
Sodium	177 mg
Phosphorus	7 mg
Potassium	50 mg

Directions

- Thoroughly wash the cucumbers & drain/pat dry.
- Leave the cucumbers whole, if small. If they're larger than the thumb, then cut them lengthwise in half.

- Place and combine well with salt in a ceramic bowl.
- Let it sit for 24 hrs. (No need to refrigerate).
- Rinse and drain the juices quickly & dry the cucumbers. Either directly put into jars, fill 3-quarters full, or place them into one large jar or crock of glass, leaving a space of 2 inches between the cucumbers & the container top.
- The tarragon & the mustard seeds are added.
- Top with at least 1-inch of white wine vinegar above the cucumbers.
- Cover the jars and leave them for 3-4 weeks in a cool place.

26. Creamy Basil Vinaigrette Dressing

6 Servings

Ingredients
- 1/2 cup of olive oil
- 1/4 cup of red wine vinegar
- 1/4 tsp ground pepper
- 1 tbsp. fresh basil
- 1 pressed clove garlic
- 2 tsps. granulated sugar

Nutrition Per Serving

Calories	49 kcals
Protein	0 g
Sodium	1 mg
Phosphorus	1 mg
Potassium	4 mg

Directions
- In a blender, combine all the ingredients.
- Puree till smooth.

27. Creamy Pasta Salad

8 Servings

Ingredients
- 1/2 tsp. celery seed
- 8 ounces med shells pasta
- 1 tsp. onion powder
- 1/2 cup of mayonnaise
- 2 tbsps. carrot, grated.
- 1/8 tsp. ground mustard
- 1/2 cup of sour cream

- 1 chopped stalk celery
- 1/4 cup of chopped Pickles

Nutrition Per Serving

Calories	188 kcals
Protein	4 g
Sodium	134 mg
Phosphorus	56 mg
Potassium	90 mg

Directions

- Cook pasta & rinse with cold water per package instructions; set aside.
- Use a whisk to mix the sour cream, celery seed, mayonnaise dressing, onion powder & ground mustard in a separate bowl.
- To cooked pasta, add the dressing.
- Mix the chopped pickles.
- Garnish it with carrot & celery.

28. Creamy Strawberry Snacks

3 Servings

Ingredients

- 3 med strawberries or other fruit
- 12 RITZ low-sodium crackers
- 1/4 cup of whipped cream cheese spread of mixed berry.

Nutrition Per Serving

Calories	134 kcals
Protein	2 g
Sodium	81 mg
Phosphorus	3 mg
Dietary Fiber	6 g
Potassium	18 mg

Directions

- Spread every cracker with cream cheese spread (1 tsp).
- Top with fruit piece or strawberry.
- Serve immediately.

29. Curried Kale

4 Servings

Ingredients

- 1 tbsp. Oil
- 4 cups Lacinato/ other kale, lengthwise sliced & then chopped.
- 1 tsp graham marsala or curry powder
- ½ sliced yellow onion.
- 1/2 cup of water/low sodium broth
- 1 tsp turmeric
- 1/4 cup of rice vinegar
- 2 tbsps. sesame seeds

Nutrition Per Serving

Calories	150 cal
Protein	3 g
Sodium	230 mg
Dietary Fiber	3 g
Potassium	30 mg

Directions
- Wash kale & cut out the tough center. Then cut crosswise nearly every 3 inches into long strips.
- Sauté the onion until translucent in the oil. Add the curry powder & turmeric and let them roast for a min or so.
- Add the kale and the chicken broth or water. Cover & watch. Then add 1/4 cup of water if it needs extra liquid.
- Keep covered & stir until the kale starts to turn bright green & wilts occasionally. Don't overcook, and it's going to turn dark.
- Remove the kale from the pan, leaving behind the juices.
- Add sesame seeds, rice vinegar, and soy sauce. Stir until the sauce becomes thick and the sesame seeds begin to pop.
- Stir in the sesame oil, & then pour over the kale & serve.

30. Dilled Carrots

Servings 6
Ingredients
- 1/2 cup plain rice vinegar
- 1 lb. carrots
- 2 tsps. Dill weed.
- 2 tsps. fresh garlic or garlic powder
- 1 1/2 cups of white vinegar
- 3 tbsps. Sugar
- 1/4 tsp. pepper

Nutrition Per Serving

Calories	58 kcals
Protein	1 g
Sodium	56 mg
Phosphorus	28 mg
Potassium	246 mg

Directions
- In small strips, Cut the carrots.
- Steam in the microwave for about 3 - 5 minutes.
- Cool by plunging the carrots into ice water.
- Now Mix all the other ingredients.
- Pour over the carrots.
- Now Place in some covered container & chill overnight.

31. Easy Chicken Pot Pie

8 servings

Ingredients
- 3 tbsp. Flour
- 1 package of Pillsbury Pie Crust
- 3 cups of Water
- 3 tbsp. Butter, Unsalted
- 1/2 lb. chopped Mushroom
- 1/2 cup chopped Onion
- Optional: 1/4 cup White Wine
- 3 cups Mixed Vegetables, fixed
- 1 baking potato, Medium
- 3 cups Cooked turkey, chicken, or beef
- 2-3 tbsp. chopped Fresh Sage
- 1/2 cup chopped fresh Parsley

Nutrition Per Serving

Calories	316 cal
Protein	13 g
Sodium	249 mg
Phosphorus	169 mg
Potassium	468 mg

Directions
- Preheat the oven to 350° F.
- Microwave the potato for 5 to 7 minutes. Dice, peel and put aside.

- Melt the butter on a medium-high flame and brown the mushrooms and onions in a large skillet.
- Reduce the flame to medium, then add the flour.
- For 3 minutes, stir.
- Add water slowly.
- Till it thickens, stir.
- Remove from the flame.
- Mix in: Herbs, meat, and vegetables.
- In the pie pan, put 1 crust, add the filling, and cover with the 2nd crust.
- Press the sides together with a fork.
- Bake for 30 to 40 mins.

32. Easy Deviled Eggs

12 servings
Ingredients
- 1/4 cup mayonnaise
- 12 eggs, large
- For garnish: Paprika
- 1 tsp. yellow mustard

Nutrition Per Serving

Calories	110 cal
Protein	6 g
Sodium	92 mg
Phosphorus	86 mg
Potassium	64 mg

Directions
- Put the eggs and bring them to a boil in a pot of water.
- Boil eggs for almost 15 minutes, till hard-boiled.
- Drain the eggs and let them cool.
- Peel the eggshells and lengthwise cut the eggs into two.
- Remove its yolks and mash till crumbly in a mixing bowl.
- Mix the mustard and mayonnaise with the yolks.
- Spoon the mixture into each white egg, then sprinkle for additional color with paprika.
- Before serving, put in the fridge and cool.

33. Easy Pizza Sauce

Sauce for 12-inch pizza servings

Ingredients
- 1-2 tbsp. olive oil
- 1 can tomato paste (6 oz.)
- 1 tsp. dried parsley
- 1 tsp. dried oregano
- 2-3 tbsp. water
- 1-2 tbsp. fresh basil

Nutrition Per Serving

Calories	68 cal
Protein	1 g
Sodium	131 mg
Phosphorus	2 mg
Potassium	409 mg

Directions
- Mix all the ingredients together, then add a bit of water at a time till you've a fine spreadable consistency.
- Spread on the top of 2 pizzas, then add the toppings.

34. Edamole Spread

6 servings (2 1/2 tbsp. each)

Ingredients
- 3 tbsp. water
- 3/4 cup shelled, frozen green soybeans, thawed
- 1 tbsp. grated finely lemon rind
- 2 tbsp. olive oil
- 1/4 cup of parsley leaves
- 1 tbsp. lemon juice
- 1 halved garlic clove
- Optional: 1/4 tsp. tabasco or hot sauce

Nutrition Per Serving

Calories	74 cal
Protein	3 g
Sodium	5 mg
Phosphorus	38 mg
Dietary Fiber	6 g
Potassium	142 mg

Directions
- Mix all the ingredients in a blender or food processor and continue till smooth.

- Cover it and cool.
- Serve with pita wedges or tortilla chips.

35. Fajita Flavor Marinade

15 servings

Ingredients
- juice from one orange
- 1 finely diced jalapeño
- juice from one grapefruit
- 3 tbsp. vegetable oil
- 2 crushed cloves garlic, or 1/4 tsp. dried
- juice from two limes

Nutrition Per Serving

Calories	33 cal
Protein	0 g
Sodium	0 mg
Phosphorus	5 mg
Potassium	42 mg

Directions
- Mix all the ingredients together in a small bowl.
- Spillover the vegetables or the meat to coat.
- Soak for almost 1 hour before grilling, pan-frying, or barbequing.

36. Ferocious Barbecue Sauce, Low Sodium

16 servings

Ingredients
- 1/4 (6 oz.) can water
- 1 (6 oz.) can tomato paste, low-salt
- 1/2 cup minced, sauteed onion
- 1/4 cup of dark molasses
- 2 tbsp. brown sugar
- 1/8 cup of wine vinegar
- 1 tbsp. mustard
- 1 tbsp. Worcestershire sauce
- 1 1/2 tsp. barbecue spice
- 1 tsp. lemon juice

Nutrition Per Serving

Calories	34 cal
Protein	0 g
Sodium	53 mg
Phosphorus	2 mg
Potassium	214 mg

Directions
- Mix all the ingredients and whisk over a low flame in a saucepan for 15 minutes.
- It can be refrigerated for a maximum of 2 weeks.

37. Fiona's Sauteed Fresh Greens

2 servings

Ingredients
- 1 tbsp. olive oil
- 4 cups greens-mustard, packed, kale, collard, or mixed
- 1/4 tsp. ground turmeric
- 1 cup onion, thin sliced
- 1 tbsp. soy sauce, low sodium
- 1/2 tsp. sugar
- For garnish: 1/4-1/2 tsp. sesame oil and sesame seeds
- 1/2 cup rice vinegar or white wine

Nutrition Per Serving

Calories	123 cal
Protein	3 g
Sodium	283 mg
Phosphorus	35 mg
Potassium	220 mg

Directions
- Cut the greens into long shreds of 2".
- Heat the oil in the wok.
- Sauté the onion for about 2 minutes till it is translucent.
- Sprinkle the turmeric over the onions.
- Mix in sugar and cover.
- Reduce the flame and let the greens steam till tender in their juices for 5 to 8 minutes approximately. (Uncover and occasionally flip during this time. If sticky, add a bit of water)
- Remove the greens with a slotted spoon, leaving the juices in the pan.
- Add the wine and soy sauce, and heat to a boil.

- Remove from the pan and spill the sauce over the greens, when the sauce has thickened marginally, and serve.
- Garnish with seeds and sesame oil.

38. Ice and Fire Watermelon Salsa

6 servings

Ingredients
- 1 cup chopped green bell pepper
- 3 cups chopped watermelon
- 1 crushed garlic clove
- 1 tbsp. chopped cilantro
- 2 tbsp. lime juice
- 2 medium, minced and seeded jalapeño
- 1 tbsp. chopped green onion

Nutrition Per Serving

Calories	30 cal
Protein	1 g
Sodium	2 mg
Phosphorus	14 mg
Potassium	128 mg

Directions
- Mix all the ingredients until well mixed.
- Before serving, Refrigerate for almost an hour.
- This is best as a sauce or as a dip for fish or chicken.

39. Fragrant & Flavorful Basmati Rice

8 servings

Ingredients
- 1/2 tsp. ground turmeric
- 1 tbsp. butter, unsalted
- 1/2 tsp. ground cardamom
- 1 2/3 cups chicken broth, low sodium
- 1/2 tsp. ground coriander
- 1 cup of white basmati rice
- 1 minced clove garlic

Nutrition Per Serving

| Calories | 114 cal |

Protein	3 g
Sodium	25 mg
Phosphorus	13 mg
Potassium	49 mg

Directions
- Heat the butter over medium flame in a large skillet.
- Add the garlic and spices.
- Sauté for at least a minute.
- Add the rice and mix till coated with spices and butter.
- Add the chicken broth.
- Boil, then reduce the flame to medium-low.
- Cover and cook for at least 15 minutes.

40. Fruit & Herb Vinegars

2 tablespoons servings

Ingredients
- 1/2 cup berries or fruit, sliced in 1/2" pieces
- 1-quart vinegar bottle, for example, white, cider, white, or red wine
- Old salad recycled dressing jars or bottles
- 3-4 sprigs of herbs, fresh, of your choice

Directions
- Pour approximately half a cup of vinegar out of the bottle.
- Wash the fruit and prepare it. We just have to fit it in the bottle, so slice the pieces about 1/2 inch. Just transfer them in the bottle top for tiny fruits, such as blackberries or blueberries. You can try Mandarin, Orange, Lemon Grass, Italian Plum, Tarragon, or Kiwi. Try any variety you want. Blackberry Vinegar is a perfect mix with vanilla beans. Try basil, onion, sage, garlic, thyme, or leek for the savory vinegar. Try to hold the amount to around 1/2 cup of herbs and fruits per quart of vinegar, regardless of what variations you might think of.
- Put the cap on and let it stay for almost one month at room temperature.
- Use a jelly bag, cheesecloth, or strainer to strain the vinegar.
- Pour in jars, then add new herbal sprigs or some fresh fruits, paste on a nice label. Create several recipe cards with fruit vinegar ideas.
- Store it for up to one year at room temp or refrigerate it.

41. Fruit Vinegar Salad Dressing

Serving is 2 tablespoons servings

Ingredients

- 1 tbsp. poppy seeds
- 2 tbsp. sesame seeds
- 1/3 cup thinly sliced green onions
- 1/4 cup berry or fruit vinegar
- 2 tbsp. olive oil
- 1/4 tsp. paprika
- 2 tbsp. sugar

Nutrition Per Serving

Calories	130 cal
Protein	1 g
Sodium	3 mg
Phosphorus	45 mg
Potassium	77 mg

Directions
- Heat the poppy seeds and sesame in the oil till the seeds are golden for almost 5 minutes.
- Cool them.
- Mix sugar, vinegar, and paprika till the sugar dissolves.
- Add the cooled oil with the green onions and the seeds.
- Serve it over salad.

42. Garlic-Herb Seasoning

4 servings

Ingredients
- 1 tsp. Basil
- 2 tsp. Garlic powder
- 1 tsp. Powdered lemon rind
- 1 tsp. Oregano

Nutrition Per Serving

Calories	12 cal
Protein	0 g
Sodium	1 mg
Phosphorus	16 mg
Potassium	47 mg

Directions
- Combine all the ingredients in a blender and mix well.
- Store them in a sealed container with some rice grains to avoid clumping.

43. Gingerbread

2 servings

Ingredients

- 2 tbsp. sugar
- 1 cup of Master Mix
- 1/4 tsp. ginger
- 1/4 tsp. cinnamon
- 1 egg
- 1/4 tsp. cloves
- 1/4 cup water
- 1/4 cup molasses

Nutrition Per Serving

Calories	60 cal
Protein	7 g
Sodium	30 mg
Dietary Fiber	4 g
Potassium	100 mg

Directions

- Preheat the oven to 350°F.
- Stir the spices and sugar into the mix.
- Combine the molasses, water, and egg.
- Add the liquid (half) into the mix, then beat for about 2 minutes.
- Add in the remaining liquid, then beat for a minute.
- Bake in the bread pan, lined with wax paper, for about 40 minutes. It makes a 4×6 cake.

44. Gobi Curry

4 servings

Ingredients

- 1/2 medium, finely chopped yellow onion
- 2 tbsp. butter, unsalted
- 1/2 tsp. turmeric
- 1 tsp. minced fresh ginger
- 1 tsp. garam masala
- 1 tbsp. water
- Optional: 1/8 tsp. cayenne pepper
- 1/2 cup green peas, frozen
- 2 cups of cauliflower florets

Nutrition Per Serving

Calories	58 cal
Protein	2 g
Sodium	25 mg
Phosphorus	27 mg
Potassium	152 mg

Directions

- Heat the butter over medium flame in a medium saucepan, then add the onions and cook till caramelized (lightly browned and soft).
- Add in turmeric, ginger, garam masala, and cayenne pepper.
- Stir in peas and cauliflower.
- Add the water, cover.
- Reduce the flame to low, then steam for about 10 minutes.

45. Green Beans with Dried Cranberries and Hazelnuts

8 servings

Ingredients

- 1/2 cup of hazelnuts
- 1 1/2 lb. fresh or frozen green beans
- 1/2 tsp. lemon zest
- 3 tbsp. olive oil
- 12 cups water
- 1/2 cup cranberries, dried
- 1/3 cup thinly sliced shallots

Nutrition Per Serving

Calories	199 cal
Protein	4 g
Sodium	19 mg
Phosphorus	73 mg
Potassium	246 mg

Directions

- Preheat the oven to 350°.
- Spread the hazelnuts on the baking sheet in a single layer. Bake at 350 ° for 10 to15 minutes or flip once before the skin starts to split.
- To extract the skins, move the toasted nuts to a dish or colander and wipe with a towel briskly. Chop the nuts coarsely.

- In a large saucepan, bring the 12 water cups to a boil. Add the beans and simmer for 4 minutes or till tender. Drain and immerse into the ice water. Drain, then pat the beans dry.
- Over medium flame, heat a large skillet. To the pan, add the oil, then swirl to coat. Add the shallots and cook till lightly browned. Add the beans, simmer for 3 minutes or till cooked completely, stirring sometimes. Add the hazelnuts and cranberries and simmer for one minute. Sprinkle with the lemon zest.

46. Honey Lemon Dressing

8 servings

Ingredients
- 3 tbsp. lemon juice
- 1/4 cup of honey
- 1/2 tsp. red pepper flakes, crushed
- 1/2 tsp. dried basil
- 2 tbsp. vegetable oil

Nutrition Per Serving

Calories	40 cal
Protein	<1 g
Sodium	1 mg
Phosphorus	2 mg
Potassium	31 mg

Directions

Mix together all the ingredients till well blended in a small bowl.

47. Hundred Combinations Vinaigrette

2 tablespoons serving

Ingredients
- 1/2 or 2/3 cup vinegar or lemon juice (balsamic, white, cider, red wine, raspberry, etc.)
- 1/2 or 2/3 cup oil (hazelnut, olive, avocado, canola)
- 1 tbsp. mayonnaise
- 2 tbsp. fresh herb (tarragon, parsley, thyme, basil etc.)

Nutrition Per Serving

Calories	120 cal
Protein	trace
Sodium	trace

Phosphorus	trace
Dietary Fiber	trace
Potassium	trace

Directions
- Choose one vinegar, one oil, one fresh herb, or one or two different options.
- Combine with the mayonnaise and place in a bottle.
- It can last for several weeks if refrigerated. Before serving, you might require to set out at room temp. before utilizing for the oil to liquefy.
- Options: 1 to 2 tsp. Honey, 1 tsp. Prepared mustard, 1 clove garlic (minced), 1 tbsp. Grated parmesan, 1 tsp. Minced onion or celery seed, dried oregano, curry powder, fresh black pepper (ground), or 1 tbsp. Mayonnaise. The emulsifiers within will keep the dressing of the salad from separating.

48. John's BBQ Sauce

6 servings

Ingredients
- 1/4 cup of Worcestershire sauce
- 3/4 cup of brown sugar
- 2 tbsp. canola oil
- 1/8 tsp. ground black pepper
- 1/4 cup of rice wine or other white vinegar
- 3/4 cup ketchup, no-salt-added
- 2 tbsp. mustard
- 1/2 tsp. onion powder
- 1/2 tsp. garlic powder

Nutrition Per Serving
Calories	46 cal
Protein	0 g
Sodium	102 mg
Phosphorus	8 mg
Potassium	56 mg

Directions
- Mix all the ingredients together till well blended.
- Use it immediately, or it can be stored in the fridge for up to two weeks.

49. Microwave Lemon Curd

16 Servings

Ingredients
- 3 eggs
- 1/2 cup melted butter
- 1 cup sugar, granulated
- 3 zested lemons
- 2/3 cup lemon juice, fresh
- 1/2 cup of pomegranate seeds

Nutrition Per Serving

Calories	115 kcals
Protein	1 g
Sodium	54 mg
Phosphorus	20 mg
Potassium	28 mg

Directions
- Put sugar and eggs in a microwave-safe bowl and whisk until smooth.
- Add the lemon juice, butter, and lemon zest and stir.
- Cook the mixture in a microwave at one-minute intervals and stir thoroughly at each interval. Do this until the mixture is thick enough to coat the back of a teaspoon.
- Remove the bowl from the microwave and store in sterile jars.
- You can store it for up to 3 weeks inside a refrigerator.

50. Oven Blasted Vegetables

4-6 servings

Ingredients
- 3/4 cup of carrots
- 1 Yukon gold potato
- 1 yam
- 1 onion
- 2 tbsp. olive oil
- 1 beet
- Parmesan cheese (to taste)
- 1/4 cup of fruit vinegar

Nutrition Per Serving

Calories	247 kcal
Protein	5 g
Sodium	62 mg
Phosphorus	67 mg
Potassium	243 mg

Directions
- Cut all the vegetables in equal-sized pieces and similar shapes.
- Set the oven to 500° C, and heat oil in a flat metal pan for 2 minutes.
- After adding the cut onions, potatoes, and carrots, cook it for 10 minutes.
- Stir the mixture, and after cooking for 5 more minutes, add yam and beet. Cook it for 20 minutes stirring every 10 minutes.
- Remove from oven, top it with vinegar and grated parmesan.
- Oven-Blasted Vegetables are ready to be served.

51. Pancakes with Master Mix

5 servings
Ingredients
- 1 tbsp. sugar
- 2 1/4 cups of Master Mix
- 1 1/2 cups milk
- 1 beaten egg

Nutrition Per Serving
Calories	348 kcal
Protein	9 g
Sodium	302 mg
Phosphorus	175 mg
Dietary Fiber	19 g
Potassium	260 mg

Directions
- Add sugar and Master-Mix in a medium bowl.
- In a small bowl, combine egg and milk and add both mixtures to dry ingredients at once.
- Blend thoroughly.
- Leave the mixture for 5-10 minutes.
- Oil a hot grill and cook it for 3-4 minutes until browned on both sides.

52. Pita Wedges

8 servings

Ingredients

- Margarine, butter, oil, or mayonnaise to cover the rounds
- 4 rounds of pita bread
- 1 tsp. dried oregano
- 1/2 cup fresh grated, parmesan cheese

Nutrition Per Serving

Calories	104 cal
Protein	3 g
Sodium	161 mg
Phosphorus	45 mg
Potassium	30 mg

Directions

- Spread the pita breads with a small amount of margarine, butter, or mayonnaise using a brush or paper towel, or spray it with cooking oil.
- On each round of bread, sprinkle about 2 tbs of dried herbs and parmesan cheese.
- Cut all 4 rounds into 8 sections each. (32 pieces)
- In a 450° toast the bread for 3-5 minutes, until the chips toast and the cheese melts.
- Serve with any low sodium salsas and dips like Edamole's spread or Joyce's Dip.

53. Quick Dip

8 servings

Ingredients

- 1 tbsp. and 1 tsp. Mrs. Dash (any flavor)
- 8 oz. sour cream

Nutrition Per Serving

Calories	60 cal
Protein	1 g
Sodium	13 mg
Phosphorus	20 mg
Potassium	35 mg

Directions

- Using a fork, mix Mrs. Dash and sour cream until well blended.
- Let sit overnight

54. Quick Pesto

6-8 servings

Ingredients
- 1 garlic clove
- 2/3 cup of olive oil
- 40 basil leaves, fresh
- 10 tbsp. parmesan cheese, grated
- 2 tbsp. walnuts

Nutrition Per Serving

Calories	334 kcal
Protein	4 g
Sodium	113 mg
Phosphorus	87 mg
Potassium	47 mg

Directions
- Put all the ingredients except oil in a food processor or a blender, and process until fine
- With the processor still running, slowly add oil until everything is well blended.
- Enjoy the hot pasta.

55. Quick Mushroom Broth

2-4 servings (1 cup)

Ingredients
- 2-4 cups of water
- 5-8 mushrooms, dried
- 1/2 cup chopped celery or carrots
- 1/2 cup chopped onions

Nutrition Per Serving

Calories	24 cal
Protein	1 g
Sodium	20 mg
Phosphorus	8 mg
Potassium	62 mg

Directions
- Add all the ingredients in a saucepan and heat to boiling. Reduce the heat and let simmer for about 10 mins
- Remove from heat, strain, and it's ready.

- You can use it in any recipe that calls for chicken or beef broth

56. Healthy Chicken Nuggets

4 servings

Ingredients

- 1 cup of panko bread crumbs
- 1/4 cup of Dijon mustard
- 2 cubed, skinless, boneless chicken breasts

Nutrition Per Serving

Calories	247 cal
Protein	31 g
Sodium	484 mg
Phosphorus	284 mg
Dietary Fiber	3 g
Potassium	384 mg

Directions

- Preheat the oven to 500° F.
- Pat the chicken dry, then cube into tiny bite-size pieces of nuggets.
- After dredging into mustard, roll the pieces in bread crumbs.
- Bake the nuggets for 15 mins on a baking sheet.

Conclusion

One that is deficient in phosphorous, protein, and sodium is a renal diet. The body of an individual is different, so each patient needs to collaborate with a renal dietitian to create a diet customized to the patient's needs. A renal diet often highlights the value of eating high-quality protein and limiting the liquids.

For patients with renal failure, too much salt may be dangerous since their kidneys cannot properly remove extra fluid and sodium from the body. As fluid and sodium build up in the bloodstream and tissues, they can cause Edema, heart failure, high blood pressure, etc. Therefore, individuals with kidney disease must follow a kidney friendly diet to enjoy a healthy life.

CPSIA information can be obtained
at www.ICGtesting.com
Printed in the USA
LVHW060126220221
679596LV00030B/1532

9 781801 822398